Making a Spinet by Traditional Methods

John Barnes

Published by
John Barnes
Edinburgh, Scotland UK

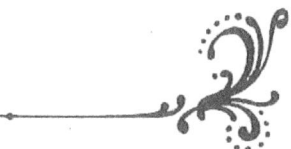

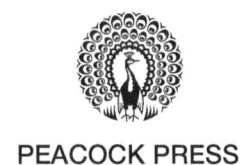

PEACOCK PRESS

Making a Spinet by Traditional Methods

John Barnes

Published by
John Barnes
Edinburgh, Scotland UK

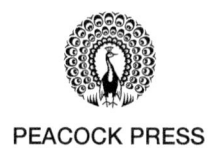

PEACOCK PRESS

© John Barnes 1985
First published 1985
Reprinted 1987
Revised 1998
Revised 2015

All rights reserved. No part of this publication may be reproduced, stored in a retrieval system or transmitted in any form or by any means, electronic, mechanical, photocopying, recordering or otherwise without prior permission of the Publishers.

Published by Peacock Press
Scout Bottom Farm
Mytholmroyd
Hebden Bridge HX7 5JS (UK)
Tel: 01422 882751
Fax: 01422 886157
www.northernbeebooks.co.uk

ISBN 978-1-908904-74-4

Cover: General view of Keene and Brackley spinet after restoration by Malcolm Ros

Design and artwork, D&P Design and Print
Printed by Lightning Source (UK)

CONTENTS

Materials	iv
Introduction	1
Bentside and Baseboard	5
Basic Structure	9
Case Sides	14
Keyboard	17
Soundboard	25
Jacks	31
Stringing and Quilling	39
Further Reading	49
Suppliers	50
Photographs	50
Index	51

MATERIALS

Part	Original	Suitable alternatives
Back, baseboard, braces, keys, keyframe, sound-bars, guide tongues	probably spruce	pine, fir, poplar
Keyboard guide rack	poplar	lime
Case sides, lid, capping for case sides, mouldings for case and lid, jack guide, keyblocks	walnut	mahogany, cherry, oak
Wrestplank, nut	beech	sycamore, maple
Jack bodies, bridge Veneers for name board, keywell and inside of case	pear	cherry or other fruitwood
Stand	oak	walnut, mahogany, cherry
Natural keyplates	ebony	stained pear
Accidental keyplates	ivory	bone, plastic, resin
Decorative keyfronts	paper	
Strings, decorative hinges and catches, bridge pins, hitch pins	brass	
Tuning pins, balance pins	iron	mild steel
Jack tongues	probably holly	beech, sycamore, maple
Quills	probably crow quill	Delrin
Soundboard	quartered European spruce	quartered sitka spruce

Introduction

READERS who use this booklet as a source of general information on the constructional methods used by makers of keyboard instruments during the seventeenth and eighteenth centuries will, I hope, find it a useful guide whether they are concerned with Italian, Flemish or other traditions. The various regional traditions have much in common. Keene's techniques were influenced by the numerous instruments imported from Flanders and Italy which he would have seen and also by the practices brought from those countries by immigrant makers who settled in London. This booklet does not pretend, however, to be a general study. It is specifically about Keene's practices as they are revealed by a detailed inspection of my own spinet made about 1715 by Stephen Keene and Charles Brackley (Boalch no. 22), supplemented by observations on two Keene instruments which I have restored. This restriction makes it possible for me to describe the techniques used in one workshop, rather than dealing in qualified generalities. It also enables the booklet to be used in conjunction with my full-sized drawing and set of photographs of the same instrument. Together they give a maker, amateur or professional, more information about the construction of this particular spinet than is currently available on any other early keyboard instrument. My intention is that the drawing should show what Keene did and the booklet should explain how, why and in what order he did it. I have not assumed any specialized knowledge of musical instrument making because I want to enable anyone with a knowledge of basic woodworking techniques and tools to make an instrument even if he has not previously done so. I have described the simplest techniques and those requiring the minimum of special tools, leaving the maker to adapt these according to the power tools available and the number of instruments he intends to make. I know from experience that the simplest ways are often elusive.

If you copy this design you will be benefitting from the mature experience of one of the finest makers of the English spinet who worked at a period when the instrument reached one of its high points. This experience was not only directed to producing a good design, but also to the efficient production of spinets in a small workshop. I have taken care that the drawing accurately reproduces the design as Keene left it, and have noted Keene's construction lines since they contain clues to his methods.

Someone coming to spinet making through modern furniture production, or through modern piano construction, will have a wealth of experience which will seem to be relevant to this task. But I would like to caution him that by the time he has followed these instructions, even to the extent of making *one* spinet, he will appreciate that Keene was a thoroughly practical man who knew how to make spinets quickly and efficiently and how to make a living at it. By all means begin with wood which has been accurately cut by modern equipment – this is something machines do well – but be sceptical of your ability to improve on Keene's methods when the instrument is being assembled. Most modern methods demand jigs and templates and lend themselves to making at least thirty identical spinets. Smaller quantities do not justify the time spent making jigs or templates. It is much more appropriate to use old methods if the aim is to produce a spinet or a few spinets in a small workshop.

Most parts of any complexity on old keyboard instruments were marked out with a knife, scriber or marking gauge and then sawn, planed or chiselled by eye. Some of the construction lines disappeared during these processes, but if they did not, there was no feeling that they should be concealed or removed, and sometimes they were incorporated into a decorative scheme (for example the two bold lines which run across the naturals just in front of the sharps on the spinet keyboard).

I do not claim to know exactly what Keene did at each stage, but I have tried to make sense of all the construction lines and to work within the harpsichord tradition as far as we know it. If you discover a better method than one I recommend here, please share it with me. But finish the spinet first, and do not go out of your way to innovate. Such an attitude wastes a lot of time.

There seem to be two rules governing the way builders like Keene set about making their instruments. The first involved the workshop patterns which served for many of the functions of a full-sized drawing. This can be stated as: *whenever possible, reduce the elements of a design to a series of linear measurements indented as graduations on a wooden ruler.* The second principle involved the order of making the parts, in which a craftsman could otherwise please himself. This can be stated as: *choose the order in which the parts are made and assembled so that the variations which inevitably occur in making the earlier parts can be compensated in the later parts.*

The first principle tended to standardize the important measurements of an instrument, such as keyplate widths and string lengths, but the second principle had the effect of introducing an element of chance into most of the less important dimensions with the later processes progressively more and more subject to random variations. A craftsman marking the nut pins according to these principles, for instance, was making sure his quills would be even in length in spite of variations in the jack positions and in the bridge-pin positions. Since the bridge-pin positions were affected by any errors in the positioning of the bridge itself, it is clear that the element of chance in the positioning of the nut pins was fairly large. The working of the two rules will become clear as we proceed with the construction.

Keene used the traditional kind of glue made from animal skins, hooves, etc. This was dissolved in hot water in a heated glue pot and brushed hot onto wood that had been warmed. When properly used it sets fairly firmly as soon as it has cooled, so that it is usually possible to proceed with the next operation almost immediately. Of course, the joints do not develop their full strength until they are dry. It is always possible to take these joints apart again by soaking them in water, which is very valuable when repairs are necessary.

If you prefer to use modern cold adhesives, some of the processes will be easier, but you may need to apply cramps until the glue is set, and if you have to take the joint apart it may not be easy.

The section headings are based on the script used on the nameboard. They were lettered by Sheila Barnes, and will help those who want to letter their own nameboards in a similar script. I have had valuable help on traditional tools and techniques from Peter Mactaggart. The photographs to which the text refers were taken by Peter Barnes. A lens is recommended when examining them for small details.

The notes names are written in the standard way for early keyboard instruments. In this system the compass of this spinet begins at GG, double capitals being used up to BB, single capitals for the next octave (C–B), while lower case letters are used for subsequent octaves, without superscript (c–b), or with superscript (c^1–b^1, c^2–b^2, c^3–e^3). In this system, middle c is written c^1.

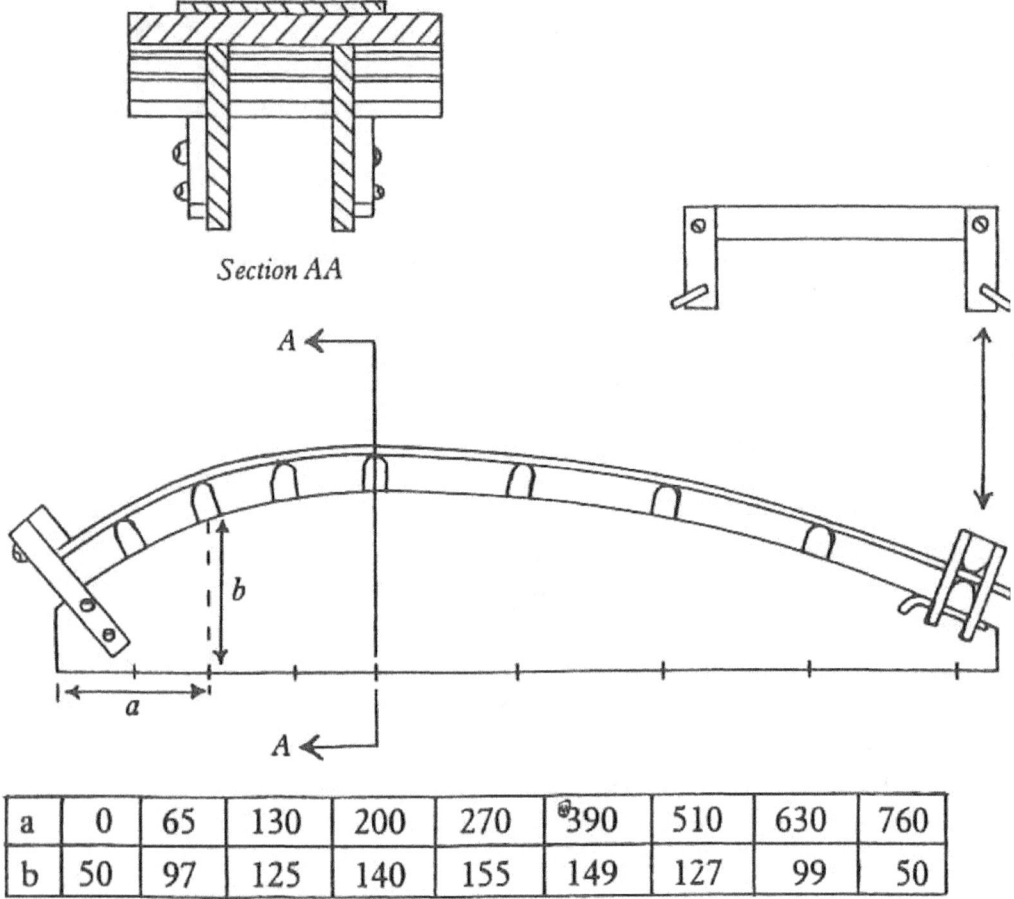

| a | 0 | 65 | 130 | 200 | 270 | 390 | 510 | 630 | 760 |
| b | 50 | 97 | 125 | 140 | 155 | 149 | 127 | 99 | 50 |

Fig. 1 Bentside bending form

Bentside and Baseboard

THE wood for the bentside should be straight grained and the grain should run parallel, or nearly parallel, with the surface so that the wood will not split when it is bent. The grain direction is less important at the end which is less curved. The thickness of the bentside varies from 8.9 mm near the tail to 7.1 mm near the keyboard, and is 8.2 mm half-way along. Presumably Keene tapered this piece because it made bending easier. The finished bentside is 750 × 176 mm, but it should be cut so that it is about 850 × 179 mm and trimmed after it is bent. A simple, easily-made bending form, with the bentside in place, is shown in figure 1. The curve is sharper than the finished bentside needs to be in order to allow for the amount the wood will spring back when it is released. The form can be adjusted by putting washers under the cross-bars or by planing the lengthwise runners to alter their shape.

This design of spinet will accommodate quite a lot of variation in the curve of the bentside, and the result will be good as long as your curve does not deviate from the original by more than about 5 mm at any point. This tolerance can be exploited provided that the bentside is made first and the baseboard is then cut out to fit it.

Hubbard records several eighteenth-century references to immersing a bentside before bending it on p. 211, while on p. 276 he provides a translation from Peter Sprengel's *Handwerk und Künste in Tabelen* of 1773 where he says that bentsides were cramped on a form after they had been immersed in water. That a similar technique was employed by the Blanchets is implied by the presence of a 'lead trough for soaking bentsides with a bending form' listed in their inventory of 1726 (Hubbard p. 291). No mention is made of heat, and it is much easier to use cold water. If the walnut bentside is soaked for 24 hours it will take up water to the extent of about 30% of its dry weight. If the width is measured accurately before immersion you will be able to follow the progress of the drying while the bentside is still on the form. It is also useful to check the weight before and after bending. The water will remain near the surface, and since it is the surface layers which are stretched and compressed by bending, this is all that is required. About 48 hours drying at 15 °C and 55% relative humidity is sufficient to evaporate most of the excess water. This method will, if necessary, produce a bentside every two days from one form, which is sufficient for most people. If the bentside is removed from the form before it is fully dry, it should be left for about a week before the baseboard is marked from it, so that the remainder of the moisture can evaporate and the timber can stabilize.

If the curve is not close enough to Keene's original, the bentside can be re-soaked when it will almost straighten out again. It can be re-bent after the form is adjusted.

For the bottom of the instrument, Keene seems to have selected a board 260 mm wide by about 2.5 m long, and sawn it into three pieces as shown in figure 2. He probably left the faces of the boards in their sawn state until the base had been glued up. Assemble the boards on the bench in the positions they will occupy in the finished base and taking a pair of boards, fold them at the joint so that the edges that will be glued together lie side by side. Cramp the boards in the vice with these edges uppermost and plane the two edges at the same time. The boards will still be flat when they are glued together even if the plane is tilted slightly, but you must avoid making the edges convex or hollow along their length. If possible use a plane that is longer than 0.5 m such as a trying plane. When each of the paired edges has been planed for jointing, the baseboard should be assembled dry and marked across the joins in pencil

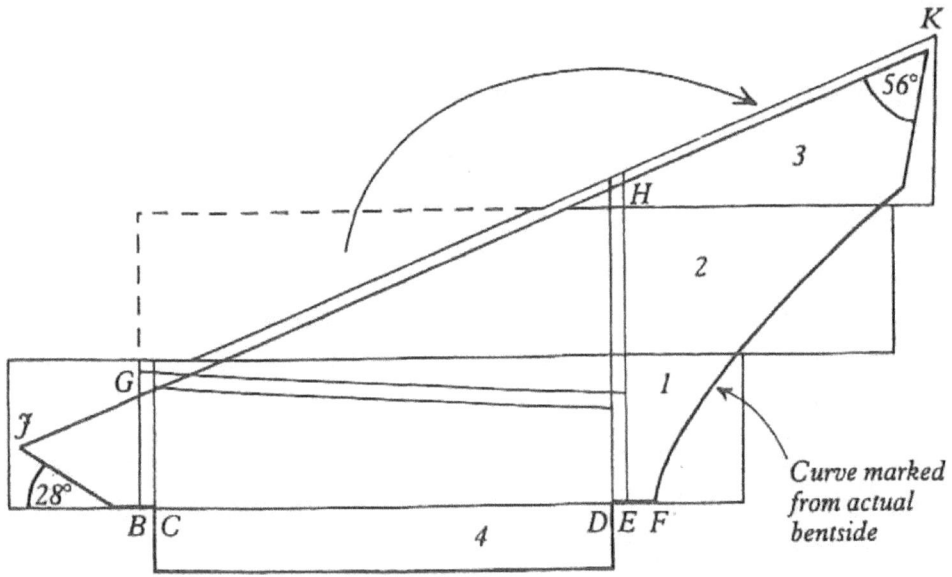

Fig. 2 Baseboard: construction and marking

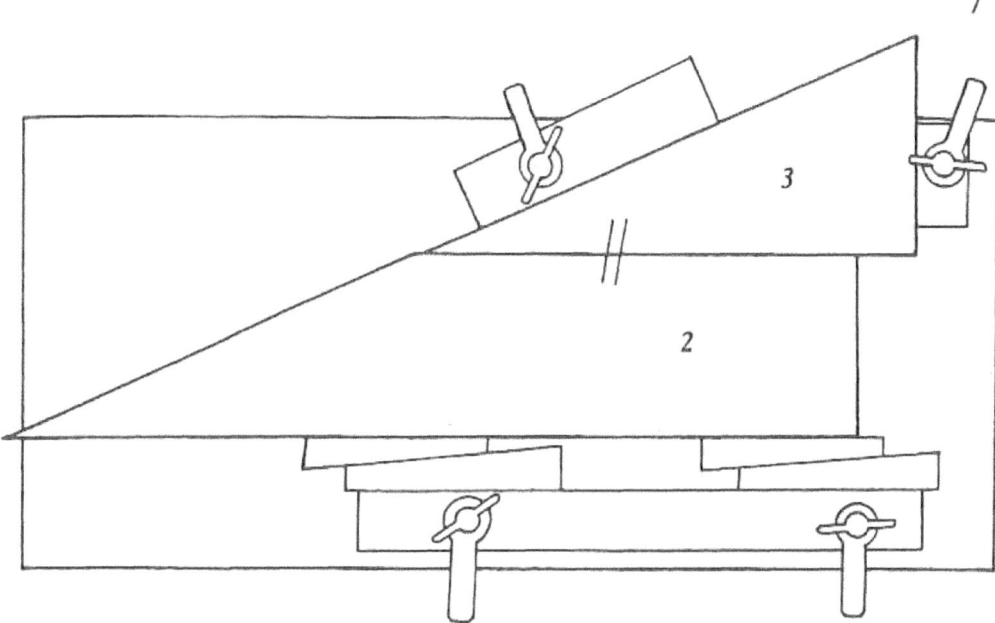

Fig. 3 Jointing the baseboard using wedges

so that the boards can be correctly placed when they are glued. The edges to be jointed are heated, spread with hot, hide glue, and rubbed together, leaving the pencil marks in line. Part 2 of the baseboard is first held vertically in the vice and part 3 jointed to it. Then part 1 is held in the vice and part 4 jointed to it. Before jointing part 4, its ends should be finished to length so that nothing needs to be done to the corners C and D. Next day the combined parts 2 & 3 and 1 & 4 are jointed to each other and the resulting unit is set aside for the joints to dry. The best way to thickness the base by hand is to plane it across the grain as then heavy cuts can be taken with little effort. If the board is left a little too thick, the last planing of each side can be along the grain to remove the roughness due to cross planing. Keene certainly used the technique of cross planing, because the underside of the keyboard of the 1668 virginal in the Russell Collection was planed across the grain leaving it slightly rough, and it was not afterwards cleaned up by planing with the grain.

The use of a planing and thicknessing machine makes it easier to thickness the whole of the 2.5 m length before cutting it into three parts. You can then glue the boards together by resting them on a horizontal surface and, if you are using modern glues, you can apply pressure with pairs of wedges as shown in figure 3.

The baseboard, jointed but not cut to shape, should then be put aside, in approximately the atmospheric conditions in which the instrument will eventually be used, until you are ready to fit the braces, wrestplank and case sides to it.

My reconstruction of Keene's scribed construction lines is shown in figure 2, BG and EH being marked perpendicular to BE. The points G and H through which the back was marked with a straight line were probably located by measuring along BG and EH. He probably also marked the rest of the outline for sawing with scribed lines, copying the bentside shape from the actual bentside he was going to use. He would have cut the straight sides with a handsaw and the bentside with a bow saw or compass saw. He would have planed the edges, using a circular plane or a spokeshave for the curve of the bentside.

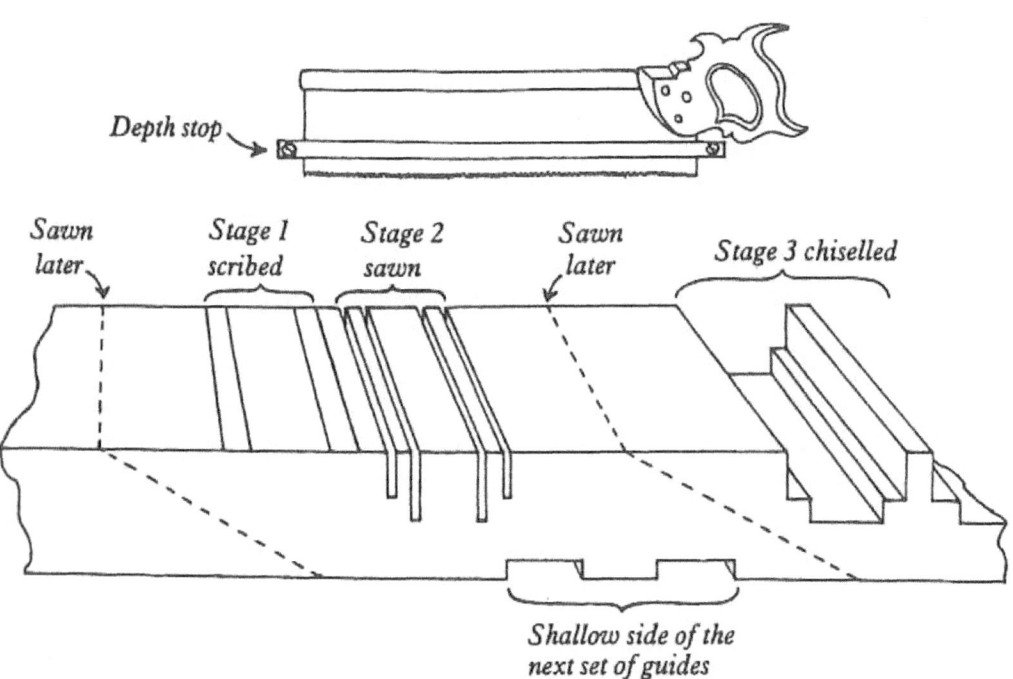

Fig. 4 Stages in making the jack guide

Basic Structure

The wrestplank is made slightly over-length and placed under the baseboard, so that it lines up at the front of the case. The ends of the wrestplank are then marked from the baseboard, sawn to length and planed.

The earliest English spinets (e.g. those by Haward and early ones by Keene) had jack guides similar to those of English virginals, but the type used in this spinet (see figure 5 and photograph 1) had become standard by the early years of the eighteenth century. It is similar to an Italian box slide but it is designed to be firmly glued to the back of the wrestplank. The slots for the jacks are formed by sawing and chiselling shallow channels in the surface of a series of rhomboid-shaped blocks, which are glued together in a line. The jack guide is finished at each end by two small triangular blocks, which in the original spinet have obviously been made from standard rhomboids since each includes the edge of a jack slot although they do not, of course, contain any jacks. Keene seems, therefore, to have made a series of standard rhomboid blocks, probably sufficient for several instruments, and then assembled them into jack guides.

Keene probably made these blocks by first preparing a number of long strips about 29 mm wide by exactly 12.3 mm thick, using the same technique of planing the strip in a groove which will be described on page 32 in connection with making jacks. These strips were probably long enough for him to cut three or four rhomboids from each one, and were probably marked across with a scriber and square, from a marked-out master strip kept as a pattern, in the way which will be described in connection with marking out the keyboard. If these scribed lines had been bold, they would have acted as convenient channels for starting the cut of a fine tenon saw in the right places. This is only a conjecture, but it works well, it is simple and quick and it is sufficiently accurate. The more conventional procedure of making knife lines and cutting by eye along the waste side of the line is much slower. The job is made easier still if the tenon saw has a strip of wood to act as a depth stop at 4.2 mm as shown in figure 4. This is the method which I recommend, but the scribed lines on the master strip must be positioned allowing for the kerf of a particular tenon saw, which should then be the only saw used with the master strip.

The depth stop automatically makes the cuts accurate in depth, which means that the wood between the pairs of sawcuts can be removed free-hand with a chisel which is about 1 mm narrower than the slot. However, all the sawcuts (including those for the tongue reliefs) should be made before using the chisel. The same tenon saw fitted with stops to give two other depths of cut (1.6 mm and 5.8 mm) can be used, along with a narrower chisel, to cut the tongue reliefs in the same jack slots. Engineers used to machining to close tolerances will be worried by the apparent crudity of these methods, but Keene's blocks were not slotted with great accuracy, and he probably knew how to get the job done easily and quickly, and with sufficient accuracy for the jacks to work nicely in their slots. The edges of his jack slots do not appear to have been cleaned up, and are as they were left by a fine saw. The bottoms could have been cut with a chisel to judge by their appearance. Consequently, I think he used methods something like those I have suggested above. The dimensions of the blocks which are shown on the full-sized detail drawing have been rationalized from measurements of many of Keene's blocks, whose individual measurements vary considerably. After sawing and chiselling all the slots in each of the strips, the strips can be sawn diagonally, as shown on the full-sized detail drawing, into individual rhomboids.

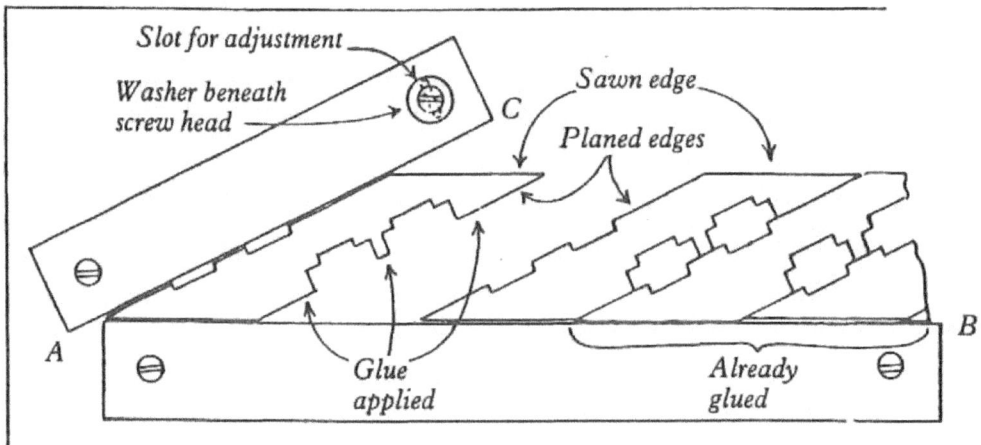

Fig. 5 Assembling the jack guide

Before gluing the blocks together to form a guide, the angle between the interfaces and the long edges must be established. There is no evidence concerning Keene's method, and what follows is my own suggestion. The distance between jacks nos. 1 and 55 on the original spinet is 742 mm, but the way we will make the keyboard allows a useful tolerance, and anything between 738 mm and 746 mm will do. The angle will depend on the exact thickness of the strips which were used to make the blocks, and by adjusting the angle one can cope with blocks which are slightly thicker or thinner than the 12.3 mm given in the detail drawing. If the blocks deviate from this measurement it is best for them all to be bigger or smaller.

Figure 5 shows a method of establishing the gluing angle for the blocks, and of gluing the blocks together using this angle. At least twenty-nine blocks should be made, and seven of these assembled dry against the edge AB. The distance between the slots for jacks nos. 1 and 13 is the octave span at the jack guide. In the original, this measures 165 mm, so the angle set by the strip AC should be adjusted to give this octave span. This distance is not the same as the octave span at the front of the keys, which is 159 mm because of the angle that the jack guide makes with the front of the keyboard, and because a sharp is missing at each end (GG♯ and e♭^{3}) while the keys in between are fanned out to keep the end keys approximately straight.

When the angle is correct for the actual thickness of the blocks, the first block is heated and hot glue applied sparingly, avoiding getting any glue into the slots for the jacks. The glued block is placed against the strip AC and the second block is placed against the first block using the edge AB to set the angle. As soon as the glue is cold its adhesion will be sufficient to slide back the two blocks together along the edge AB so that another block, heated and with glue applied, can be placed against the strip AC and added to the two blocks already glued together. This set of three blocks is then slid back and the process repeated until the seven blocks have been assembled and glued. This is the chance to check the octave span again, and if it is between 164 mm and 166 mm it is near enough because the key tails will be sawn to match the guide. If it is outside these limits, it is still possible to pull the blocks apart and start again at a slightly altered angle. When all twenty-nine blocks have been assembled a right-angle cut should be made at the bass end, copying the full-sized drawing. Part of the piece which has been cut off is glued to the treble end to complete it.

When the glued joints of the complete jack guide are dry, the edge to be glued against the wrestplank, which now consists of the sawn edges, more or less in line, of the twenty-nine blocks, should be planed. At this stage a tilt of 2° to the vertical should be introduced into the jack slots by planing more off the part of the jack guide which will go against the top of the wrestplank. The dimensions given in the detail drawing of the blocks are sufficiently oversize to allow for this planing. The 2° tilt of the slide ensures that each jack moves upwards in its guide in exactly the direction that the cloth pad of the key moves, i.e. very slightly forwards. This gives no movement between the jack foot and the cloth pad, which is important because, if the pad carries the jack foot in a different direction from that of the guide slot, the jack has a tendency to jam, particularly in this kind of jack guide.

The jack guide should also be sawn off square at the treble end, leaving the same distance between the end and the end jack slot as that shown on the drawing. The total length of the jack guide may be slightly different from that of the original shown on the drawing, but this will not matter if the middle slot is positioned according to the drawing. The guide should then be glued to the wrestplank at a height that will allow it to be planed level with the top of the wrestplank after the glue has dried. The back of the wrestplank to the left of the jack guide should be filled out to the required width with a strip of beech. Then this strip and the back face of the jack guide are planed to a common surface, square with the top. Finally the three parts of the soundboard liner are fitted along the back surface of the jack guide, along its right-hand end, and along the short piece of wrestplank which is to the right of the jack guide. Keene reinforced the glued joint between the long section of the liner and the jack guide with six nails, avoiding the slots in the jack guide. These nails were ordinary ones with heads, except the one visible in photograph 2, which is just a shaft driven in and bent over. The head of this one may have fractured as it was being driven in.

The three baseboard braces, which are to be fitted at either end and at the back of the keyboard, should now be made up and sawn to length. The double scribed lines, shown in figure 2, on the top surface of the baseboard mark the position they will occupy. A series of holes is now drilled downwards through the baseboard midway between the lines. Later, nails will be driven through these holes from underneath. Keene used two nails for the left-hand brace, five for the right-hand brace and four for the brace behind the keyboard. Heat the lower edge of the keyboard brace, apply glue to the heated surface, rub the joint and leave the brace in the position indicated by the scribed lines. Treat the other two braces in the same way. When the glue is cold turn the baseboard upside down with the braces resting on the bench and drive in the nails through the holes already drilled to reinforce the glued joints. This is probably the way the original was made.

Keene did not glue the wrestplank directly to the cross-braces that are at each end of the keyboard; instead there is a strip about 8 mm thick glued between the wrestplank and each of the braces. The underside of Keene's wrestplank was, of course, hand planed and not as accurate as a modern machined finish. By gluing two strips across the wrestplank which would follow its contours, he had two narrow spruce surfaces which were easy to trim and fit to the tops of the braces. The two joints between the strips and the braces, which have to be glued at the same time, would then fit well and would be between spruce surfaces with a common grain direction. Even if your wrestplank has a machined underside, this construction has the merit of allowing the two cross-grained joints between spruce and beech to be made separately. The above interpretation of Keene's intentions is supported by examining the glue above and below the strips. Glue has run down the sides of the braces from the bottom edge of the strips, showing that the instrument was the right way up when this gluing was done. On the other hand, glue has not run down the sides of the strips from the joint with the wrestplank. Instead it can be seen that Keene brushed glue across the wrestplank where he was going to glue the strips on, and this would obviously have been done with the wrestplank upside down. When the wrestplank has been glued to the braces, the assembly is ready for the case sides to be fitted, beginning at the back.

Case Sides

BEFORE Keene fitted the back, he must have glued the back liner to it. The evidence for this is that the liner is nailed to the back so that the nail heads show on the inside (three of these are visible in photograph 3), and some of these nails are too close to the back of the wrestplank to have been driven in after the back was fitted to the rest of the structure. Keene seems to have located the back liner, prior to gluing, with pins driven into the back at the lower edge of the liner. Three pin holes are visible, one just underneath the liner at each end and one near the middle. The liner and back were probably warmed, glue was applied to the liner, the liner rubbed to and fro a few times and left against the pins in the right place. The nails, which were previously mentioned, had probably already been driven nearly through the liner and would have then been driven home to secure the glued joint. The locating of the liner by three pins at its edge was particularly appropriate since it needs to be accurate in a vertical direction but its position would not have been critical in the horizontal direction if, as seems likely, both the back and the back liner were over-length at this stage. The most convenient time for trimming the ends of the back is after attaching it to the baseboard, braces and wrestplank. This is because the edge of the baseboard on the right, and the baseboard and wrestplank on the left, can act as guides when you are sawing these ends and shooting them with a plane.

The glued joints between the back and the assembly of baseboard, braces and wrestplank were also reinforced with nails; two were driven through the back into the wrestplank and fourteen through the back into the baseboard. The back was probably a little over-width (as well as over-length) so that, when gluing, it could be lined up with the top of the liner opposite the other liner attached to the jack guide, but overlap a little below the baseboard. This overlap would be easy to trim when all the case sides were in place.

A characteristic feature of Keene's work is a double-V mark to show the prepared face and edge of various parts. The most prominent of these marks is on the inside of the back, but the full-sized drawing also shows others — on the turnbuckle mounting, the balance rail and the back touch rail. This last can be seen above the 59 cm mark on the rule in photograph 4. Similar marks appear on his virginal of 1668.

It is difficult to tell the order in which Keene fitted the walnut sides, but there is reason to believe that he finished at the back. He probably began with the triangular piece at each end of the keyboard. These two pieces were probably cut to fit but not glued in, and the two short pieces of the case front also cut to fit, including their mitres. Each triangle was then probably glued to its neighbouring case front and each joint reinforced with several nails from the inside faces of the triangles. One of these nails is visible in photograph 3 in the recess into which the nameboard slides, level with the upper of the two horizontal lines of inlay, and there is another similar nail further down. The lower nail disappears under the pearwood veneer, proving that the veneer was applied after the instrument had been put together. The two units were then probably glued into the right-angle corners of the baseboard, with the case fronts glued to the front of the wrestplank at each end. The glued joints with the baseboard would have been reinforced with nails which were later concealed by the baseboard moulding. A strip of spruce was used to reinforce the butt joint between each triangular piece and its baseboard brace. These strips were sited just above the baseboard and glued on the keyboard side of the braces so that they also defined the width available to the keyframe. These strips were probably glued in next, followed by the narrow board of walnut along the front which carries the lock.

The bentside was probably fitted next, by preparing the mitre at the front end to fit the mitre on the right-hand case front and cutting a mitre at the tail end. The bentside would then have been glued to the treble end of the wrestplank and glued and nailed all along the baseboard curve. This procedure would have left only the tail and the corresponding piece in front of the bass end of the wrestplank still to be fitted, each of which needs to have a mitre prepared to fit the part of the case which is already glued in. The advantage of leaving these pieces until last would have been that only one mitre needs jointing in each case, the other joint being a simple overlap with the back, which would be reinforced by nails like the joints with the baseboard. The two walnut pieces would have been left to overlap the back until the glue was dry, when they could be trimmed in line with the back. An alternative procedure would be to begin with the bentside after cutting the mitres at each end, since this is the longest baseboard joint. The disadvantage is that some lateral location must be devised to avoid attaching the bentside too near the back or front. The preferred procedure automatically provides a definite lateral location for each part as it is added.

Three reinforcing corner-blocks were fitted to the original spinet inside the case. These blocks are shown on the full-sized drawing where the back meets the tail, where the tail meets the bentside, and under the treble end of the wrestplank where the bentside meets the front of the case. They are also visible in photographs 2 and 3.

Keene cut the two walnut pieces, which lie in front of the wrestplank at the bass end, from the same plank is such a way that the grain pattern runs across the joint. He did not do this across the joints at each end of the bentside, probably because he had less choice in selecting the wood for his bentside. But cutting the sides in order from one plank of wood will improve the appearance of your spinet, particularly if the wood has a prominent grain pattern.

Keene seems to have fitted the tail and bentside liners after the sides were in place, because surplus glue ran down the inside of the case in two places. One of these glue runs, which is on the tail near to the joint with the bentside, can be seen in photograph 3. The tail liner would have been fitted first, followed by the bentside liner working from the tail towards the wrestplank. Bending the bentside liner was made easy by thirteen kerfs cut from the concave edge. Keene fitted a corner block between the end of the bentside liner and the liner behind the wrestplank. The upper braces would have been fitted at this stage.

The walnut lid and flap can be cut at this stage, but it is better to make them a little oversize in the direction at right angles to the grain, and allow them several weeks to stabilize their width before finally cutting them to fit the case.

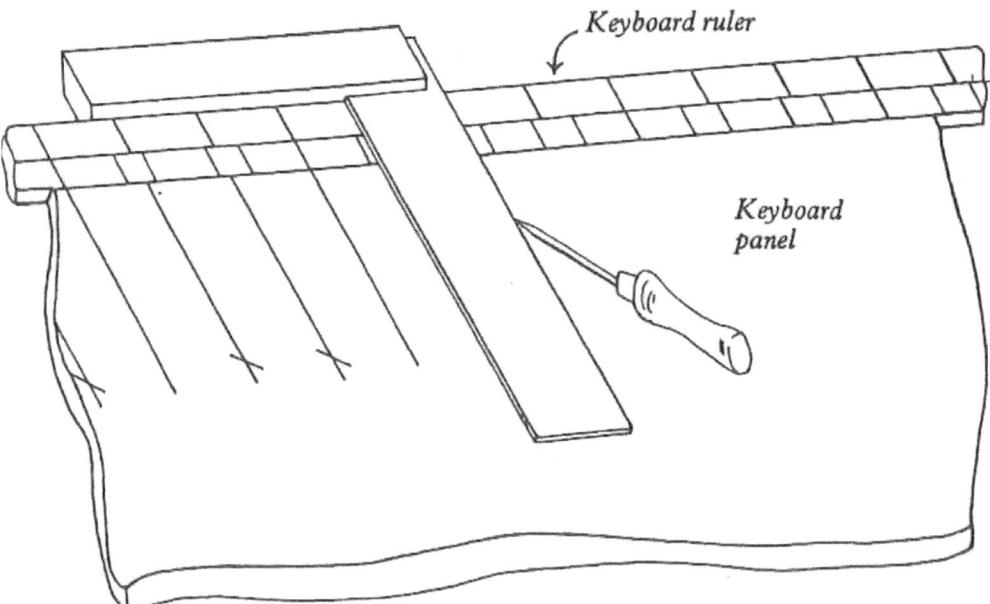

Fig. 6 Using the keyboard ruler with a square and scriber

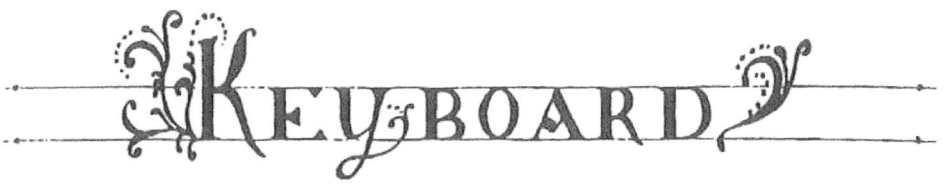

KEYBOARD

THE back member of the keyframe, the two side-pieces and the balance rail should be jointed and glued together, leaving the side-pieces slightly too wide to fit the keywell. When the glue is dry, the sides are planed until the keyframe is a good but not tight fit in the keywell. At this stage the rack and the key-blocks have not been fitted. The keyframe is held down by two turn-buttons at the front and two small blocks glued to the cross-brace which runs behind the keyboard. These are best fitted at this stage, after which the sloping shelf which runs between the top of the cross-brace and the jack-guide liner can be nailed into place.

The keyboard as it exists before the keys are sawn apart will be referred to as the 'keyboard panel'. It is made by jointing several boards of spruce with their grain running from front to back, i.e. along the individual keys. The joints are glued in the same way as those in the baseboard, and are allowed to occur at random. There is a slight tendency for the keys incorporating these joints to bend, but it is not troublesome and certainly not worth the bother of trying to get the joints to coincide with the cuts between the keys. Keene's joints occured in keys B, e^1 and $g\sharp^2$. The general practice of makers was to cover the naturals with pieces of wood which were a whole number of naturals wide – usually either two or three – so that all the joins disappeared when the keys were cut apart. However, most of the ebony which Keene used happened to be about 2½ naturals wide and therefore potentially wasteful. Keene, in fact covered the thirty-four naturals economically with thirteen pieces of ebony at the expense of leaving joins in five natural keyplates: f, d^1, b^1, g^2 and c^3. These are not very noticeable today and were no doubt almost undetectable when new. Keene made the same economy in his virginal of 1668 in the Russell Collection, Edinburgh University, which has the snakewood covering joined in the f^1 keyplate, and also in his spinet of c. 1680 in the Royal College of Music, London. This suggests that the cost of exotic hardwoods was far from negligible to Keene.

Old makers had a simple and efficient system for marking the divisions between keyplates which is explained by Dom Bedos in his *L'Art du facteur d'orgues* (1766) in connection with organ keyboards (see Hubbard pl. 38 and p. 222 for a translation of the relevant section). They constructed a keyboard ruler (Dom Bedos called it *regle du clavier*) which

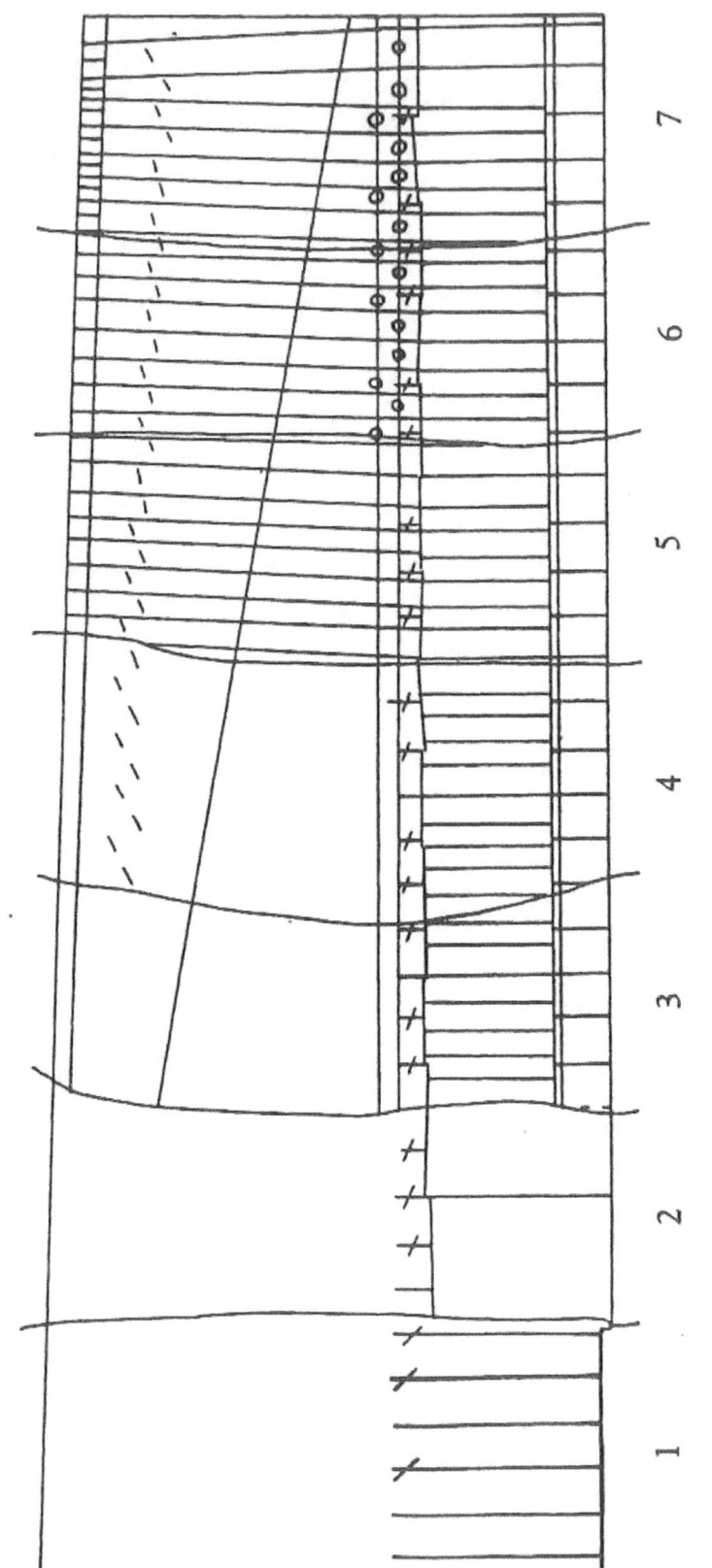

Fig. 7 Successive processes in marking the keyboard panel

indicated all the lateral divisions between the keyplates by two series of deeply scribed lines which were also inked over so that they could be easily seen. The keyboard ruler corresponding to Keene's keyboard is shown at the right-hand edge of the full-sized drawing. As shown in figure 6, this ruler was probably fixed against the front of the keyboard panel and a square and a scriber used to mark the lines on the panel. After a little practice, these lines can be marked quickly and accurately. The scribing tool is placed in one of the grooves on the ruler, the square is slid along the ruler until it touches the scriber; the square is held firmly while the scriber is lifted and brought down to make a bold scribed line against the square on the panel. The scriber is then lifted again, set into the next groove on the ruler, the square brought firmly up to it and another scribed line made on the panel. The thirty-five grooves, which correspond to the edges of the naturals, can be copied onto the panel in about 2½ minutes.

Keene's method of work on his keyboard panel is illustrated in figure 7, which is divided into seven sections showing the appearance of the panel at each of seven stages. In the first stage, the divisions between the naturals on the spruce panel were marked, and diagonal strokes were made across the divisions which corresponded to the sharps. These divisions and the diagonal strokes are visible on some of the sharps in photograph 6 (e.g. C♯ and E♭) and are very noticeable on both the BB♭ and E♭ keys which appear in photograph 4. The divisions enabled Keene to cut his prepared ebony slabs to the required widths and to glue them on in the right places, as shown in figure 7, section 2. Keene's ebony pieces were tapered from front to back to save material and weight and were probably sawn about 4.5 mm thick at the front and 2.6 mm thick at the back, judging from the thickness of his finished keyplates. When glued on they probably had a planed surface underneath and a sawn finish on top.

Section 3 shows the next stage. The top of the ebony is planed, which will be much easier if the ebony pieces are matched for the direction in which the grain rises or falls (as is mentioned on page 25 in connection with jointing the soundboard). The colour should also be matched if this varies noticeably. At this stage Keene cut the two construction lines deeply into the ebony from side to side. The front line showed where the chamfers between the naturals reached, and the rear one indicated the position of the front of the sharps. Although they were construction lines, they were cut boldly so that they formed part of the decorative effect. Then he marked the divisions between the naturals again (the marks previously made on the panel being now partly covered by the ebony), and this time he also marked the positions of the sides of the sharps. Section 3 also shows four lines scribed on the back of the panel, the first showing the line of balance pins for the naturals, the second one for the sharps, the third a diagonal identifying the key positions after the keys were separated, and the fourth a construction line showing how deep to cut the slots for the guide tongues at the ends of the keys.

Keene's method of ensuring that his key-tails lay exactly under his jacks was the standard practice throughout the sixteenth, seventeenth and eighteenth centuries. The keyboard panel was fixed temporarily to the keyframe in the correct place, probably by putting a small nail through the panel and into the balance rail at the points where the top and bottom keys were later to be pivoted. The panel would have been supported by a strip of wood where the back touch cloth was to go later, and a dummy jack was dropped into each jack slot in turn. A smart tap with a hammer made an impression of the foot of the jack in the soft wood of each key, as shown on the full-sized drawing, in figure 8 and in section 4 of figure 7. The right hand edge of many of these impressions

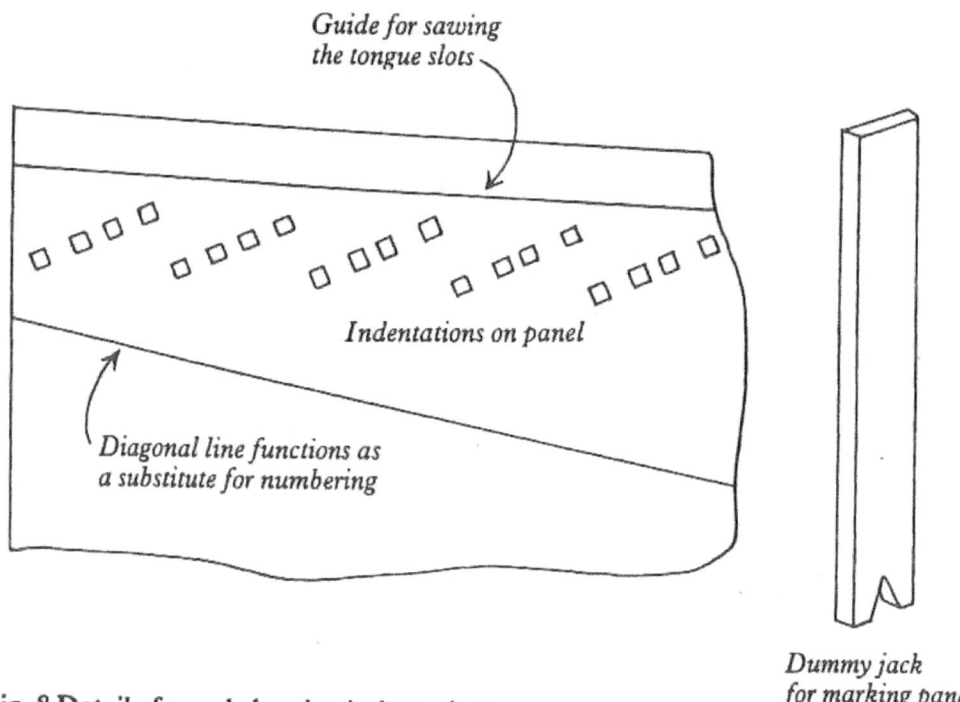

Fig. 8 Detail of panel showing indentations made by the dummy jack

can also be seen in photograph 6 and are particularly obvious on the $g\sharp^1$, a^1, c^2, e^2 and f^2 keys. Straight lines were then scribed from the lines on the ebony to the back of the panel, each one passing midway between two impressions as shown in section 5. Section 6 shows the balance-pin positions which are marked by eye with dents to start the drill in the right place. Section 7 shows the guide-tongue slots; these are cut carefully and squarely by eye with a tenon saw.

The modern maker of a spinet or a few spinets can do no better than follow these simple, quick and accurate methods of marking out. If keyboards are made in batches of more than about twenty, there may be advantages in more elaborate jigs. The maker following old methods, however, should notice that the cutting lines for the key-tails shown on the full-sized drawing are those which followed one particular jack guide made about 1715. These should *not* be followed for a new keyboard, but new positions for the key-tails must be marked out to suit the jack guide actually made for use in the new spinet. This, like the derivation of the curve of the baseboard from the actual bentside, is an example of the application of the second rule mentioned on page 2.

Before the keys are cut apart, it is necessary to ensure that after separation they remain in their former positions. This is done by drilling the balance-pin holes through the keyboard panel and into the balance rail in one operation, and by carefully copying the positions of the guide-tongue slots onto the piece of poplar from which the rack is to be made. These two operations must be done within a few hours of each other so that the width of the panel does not have time to respond to changes of humidity.

The rack is made from a piece of poplar $4.5 \times 43 \times 830$ mm. This length gives about 20 mm spare at each end, which is useful for nailing the poplar to a backing strip of oak, beech, etc., against which the chisel cuts can be made. Photographs 4 and 5 show the two gauge lines on each face marking the top and bottom of the slots which guide the tails of the keys. The first stage in making these slots is to cut a pair of parallel knife lines 1.7 mm apart for each of the fifty-six guide-tongue marks which have already been made. The easiest way of producing the pairs of lines is to make up a special square, as shown in figure 9, with a stock of hardwood which is about $120 \times 35 \times 18$ mm, and with two metal blades with a gap between them. Metal strips about $80 \times 12 \times 1$ mm are suitable, and two pieces of broken hacksaw blade could be used if necessary. The special square should be aligned with the first mark (e.g. placing the mark midway between the two blades) and a knife line cut along each of the two blade edges which form the gap. Keene evidently cut these lines towards the bottom of the rack, because they overran the lower gauge line, as would be natural for a man working for his living and wasting no time. The knife lines have, of course, disappeared except for the overruns, and these can be seen in photograph 5. The lines were cut to a depth of about 0.7 mm, which does not require much pressure with a soft material like poplar.

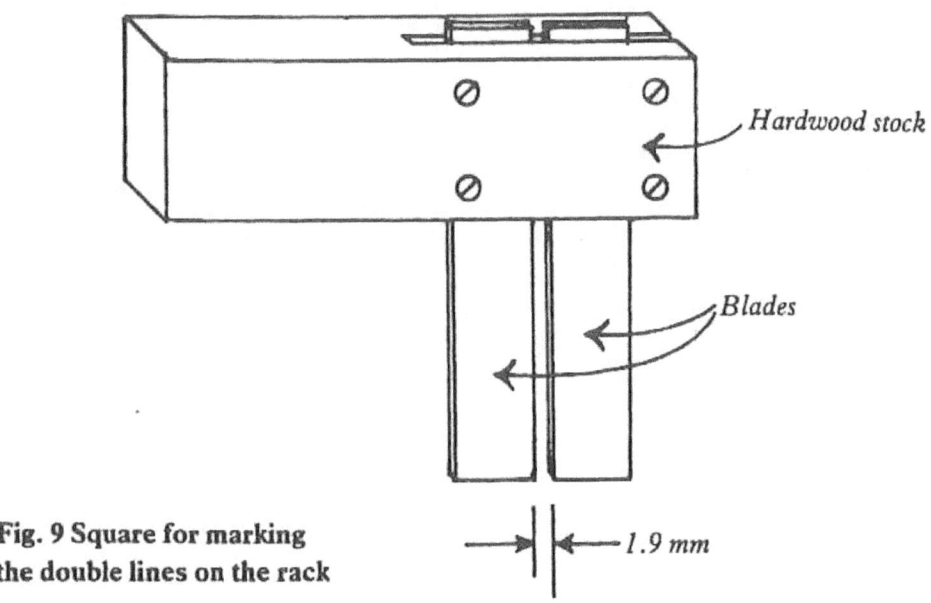

Fig. 9 Square for marking the double lines on the rack

The second stage is to open out the rack slots as shown in figure 10 by placing a 29 mm chisel in each knife line in turn and using a mallet to make it cut to a depth of about 1.5 mm. To Keene, this chisel was presumably a standard width of 1⅛ inches. It saves a little time to make the incisions on one knife line of each pair and then turn the rack and its backing strip round to incise the remaining lines. The bead of wood between the two cuts is then removed using a piece of piano wire about 0.8 mm diameter sharpened like a chisel and held in a pin vice. If the point is inserted near one of the incisions the bead can be lifted in spite of being wider than the gap on the top surface. Then the chisel can be driven another 1.5 mm into the same incisions. After removing the second bead of wood, the chisel can be driven through the poplar and into the backing, completing the cutting of the slots. In order to cut to 1.5 mm depth without producing too much pressure in the wood across the chisel slot, and to be able to cut through the rack without damaging the sides of the slots, the grinding angle of the chisel needs to be about 12°. The chisel cuts are merely reliefs, since the tongue only touches the smooth side of the knife line. The slight breakage of the back surface of the rack where Keene's chisel cut through is visible in photograph 4.

The keyframe is completed by gluing the lower edge of the rack to the back of the keyframe, inserting the balance pins (mild steel rod about 2.4 mm diameter cut to 29 mm lengths) and fixing the balance and back-touch cloth as shown in the full-sized drawing. The lateral placing of the rack must be correct, otherwise all the keys will be canted to the right or left. There are two lines on the top key which are visible in photograph 6 (below the *Fecerunt* on the nameboard) and which may have been designed to help in the placing of the rack. They were scribed perpendicular to the front of the panel before the keys were sawn apart, and were probably used to ensure that the keys were again perpendicular to the line of the keyfronts when the rack was being positioned.

Keene used red bushing cloth 1.3 mm thick and 8 mm wide for the balance cloth. He held the strip in his left hand, pressed it over the pins and cut it on the left of the pins with a knife – some of the marks where his knife cut into the balance rail are visible in photograph 7. For the back touch, Keene used several layers of woollen cloth – probably four – totalling 9.4 mm in thickness, and held taut between two tacks. The tack holes are now empty and show that the cloth has been replaced.

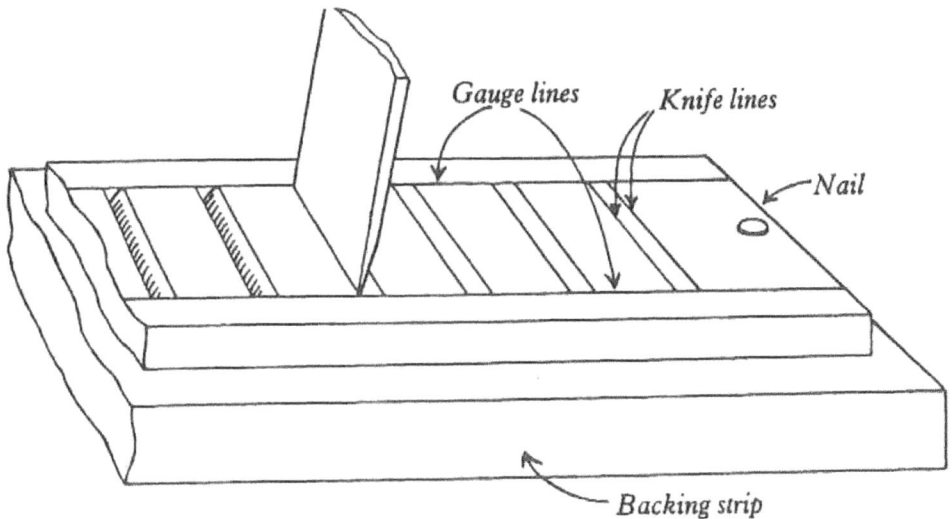

Fig. 10 Cutting the rack slots with chisel and mallet

The saw Keene used for cutting the keys in the ebony-covered part of the keyboard panel made a kerf of 1.0 mm. This is known because some of his cuts overran into the front of a sharp (see, for instance, the f♯¹ key, which is the seventh sharp from the right in photograph 8). The saw was held at about 35° to the key surface, and must have had fine teeth because

Keene chose to leave the edges of the ebony just as they were left by the saw. These cuts were made with great precision. Keene probably sawed between the tails of the keys with a frame saw or a bow saw, but nowadays these cuts are usually made with a small band-saw. The cuts from the front and back of the keyboard panel stop at the scribed line which defines the fronts of the sharps, except between keys b & c, and between e & f. As a result the panel is separated into units, mostly of five or seven keys, which hang together across the fronts of the sharps. Keene probably severed the sharps by making a chisel cut from above and below in the waste part just in front of each sharp, breaking them off at the neck formed by the chisel cuts. Alternatively, the sharps may be separated with a fret-saw. At this stage the sharps still have an ebony layer which can be removed by dipping them into hot water or by the application of a hot iron.

Keene cleaned up the saw marks on the spruce part of the keys, both naturals and sharps, slightly undercutting them as can be seen in photograph 8. He glued a patch of the same red cloth that he used for the balance washers over the mark left by the foot of the dummy jack. By applying the glue under the front and back edges of the cloth, and by leaving the centre part without glue, he avoided stiffening the cloth at the point of contact with the jack. He inserted the guide tongues in the saw cuts at the key ends without glue. Keene's method of opening up each balance hole to enable the key to rock was to insert a balance pin, probably held in a short piece of hardwood, and rock it backwards and forwards. The balance holes of keyboards by the Ruckers family were made in the same way. This method functions perfectly well although later eighteenth-century makers usually made the more elaborate rectangular balance mortices. Keene finished the naturals by rounding the sides in front of the first side-to-side score line and gluing on the decorative paper keyfronts. He applied black paint to the spruce below the ebony coverings, except where they were alongside the sharps, and painted the keyfronts at the same time. The sharps were presumably completed, after assembling all the keys on the keyframe, by gluing on the white touch plates centrally between the ebony of the naturals. Keene's sharps were ivory, probably cut as segments from the hollow part of a tusk, so that there was hardly any waste. Ivory-coloured resin need not spoil the appearance or feel of the keys; alternatively bone can be used, especially if a vertical plate of ebony is sandwiched between two bone plates, to form a 'skunk-tail' sharp, which is a contemporary style employing thinner pieces of ivory.

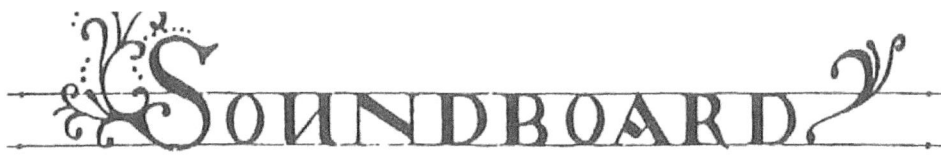

Soundboard

THE Keene and Brackley soundboard is thinner than that of the average spinet and, when one is making a copy, it helps if the separate boards are reduced in thickness until they are only a little too thick before they are jointed together. But the final thicknessing must follow the jointing process, and the necessary planing down becomes nearly impossible if adjacent boards have grain which rises in opposite directions. That is to say, it is better if the grain of all the boards is horizontal, but if the grain meets the surface at a small angle, the boards should be glued up so that the whole soundboard can be planed in one direction. In principle, the preparation of soundboard joints is the same as that of the baseboard, but the trying plane is used on its side with the pieces of soundboard parallel to the bench surface and spaced off it by a board about 20 mm thick. The longest piece of soundboard also needs to have the edge that will meet the back edge of the jack guide prepared, since this joint will be visible. The step in the soundboard at the treble end of the jack guide is formed by an extra piece 90 × 23 mm, which is designed to allow the treble end of the bridge to vibrate more freely than it would if the front edge of the soundboard were straight.

The normal woodworking bench is too narrow to support a soundboard while it is being worked on, and a firm table about 1.8 × 0.8 m with a flat solid top is required. As with the baseboard, the whole soundboard should be assembled dry from its component pieces, the pieces numbered and marked across the joints with short, pencil lines, as shown in figure 11, so that the boards can be glued together in the right relationship. If the glue used for the soundboard joints will adhere to the table top, the top should be covered with a layer of paper.

Three sides of the soundboard piece, numbered 1 on figure 11, should be cut exactly to size, leaving only the side which fits against the bentside to be cut later. Then piece 2 should be cramped near to the back edge of the table, and piece 1 glued to it. Piece 3 is placed in position in front of piece 2 and five or six pairs of wedges placed in front of piece 3 so that there is a pair of wedges about every 200 mm along the joint. A suitable board is then cramped in front of the wedges as shown in figure 11, to take their thrust. If hot glue is to be used, the jointing surfaces should be warmed e.g. by an electric radiant strip heater. Then glue should be spread on the edge of piece 3 and the two pieces rubbed to and fro a few

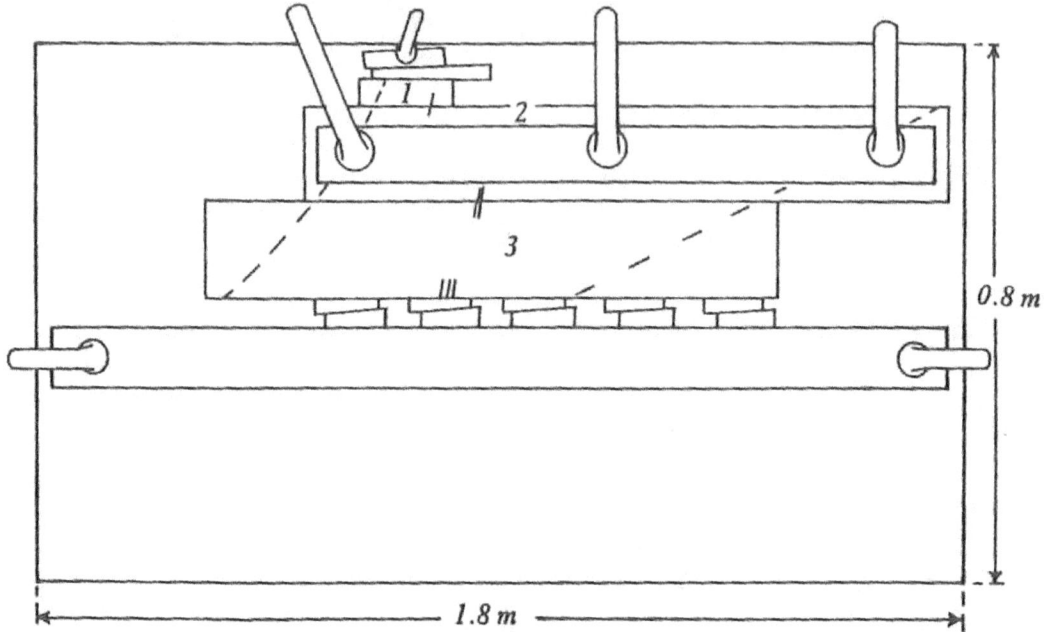

Fig. 11 Gluing the soundboard joints. The dotted lines across the soundboard pieces show the edges which are cut later.

times leaving the pencil marks in line with each other. At the same time, the two boards that are being jointed must be pressed against the table to make sure that a step is not formed at the joint. Then weights are quickly placed along the joint to prevent the boards from bowing upwards when they are cramped (tinned foods are useful as weights), and each pair of wedges tapped together with a small hammer to provide even but moderate pressure at the joint. With long joints it is an advantage to have an assistant to help with spreading the glue and with rubbing the joint. As soon as the glue is cold, soundboard piece 3 can be cramped firmly down along its whole length, e.g. with a wooden beam faced underneath with thick felt, and the board which resisted the thrust of the wedges uncramped. Then piece 4 can be glued and wedged following the procedure described above, and so on until the complete soundboard is glued together.

When the joints are dry, the soundboard should be exposed on both sides and left in a fairly dry atmosphere until its moisture content becomes approximately the same as it will be when it is glued into the case. The edges should now be cut so that the soundboard fits somewhat loosely inside the case. At this stage the inside of the case has not been veneered with pearwood. Then the soundboard should be cramped to the table and the top surface finished with a plane and, if necessary, a cabinet scraper. After this process, the soundboard is turned over and the underside is planed so that the thickness conforms to the measurements marked in the various places on the full-sized plan. The finish of the underside does not need to be as good as that of the top surface, but care should be taken not to mark the top surface during the thicknessing operations.

The device shown in figure 12 is designed to be cramped near the back of the table on which the soundboard is being prepared, so that the soundboard can be released from its cramps and slid under the hinged arm as many times as is necessary to monitor the reduction of thickness. After the rim of the dial gauge has been rotated to set the pointer to register zero when the arm rests on the table, the dial gauge will register one tenth of the thickness of the part of the soundboard which is under the metal dome. Suitable domes are made for fitting under the legs of chairs and tables. A dial gauge reading 0.5 mm or 1 mm for a complete revolution of the pointer is suitable. The weight of the arm should be sufficient to hold the soundboard flat against the table, but not so heavy that it prevents the soundboard from slipping easily under the dome.

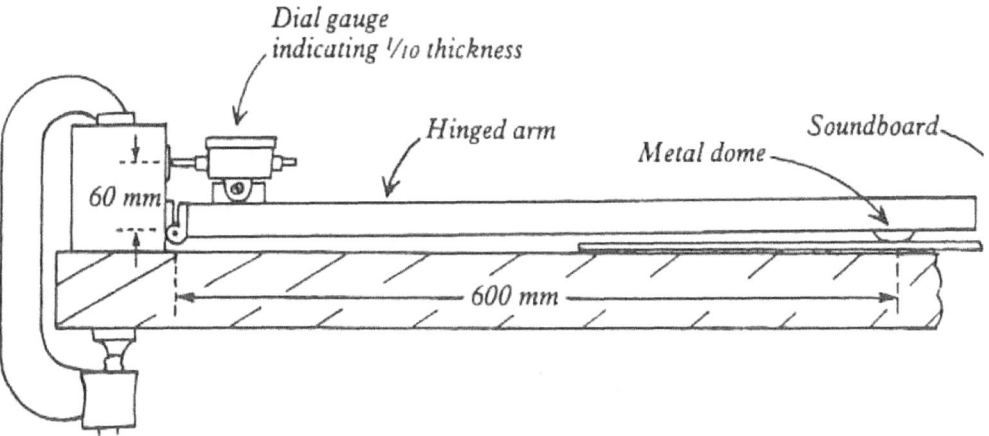

Fig. 12 Soundboard thickness measurement

Keene's bridge has a joint 55 mm from the treble end, presumably because two boards had been shot together so that several bridges could be cut from the same panel. The grain in each piece runs the same way as the join. While any bridge that is cut to shape rather than bent has the grain approximately parallel to the bridge in the bass region, it will have short grain at the treble end. The bridge therefore needs careful handling when both sides have been sawn, but the sloping side, which faces the hitch pins, can be sawn and cleaned up with a spokeshave before the cut is made that separates the bridge from the rest of the board. Keene would have used a bow saw but a band-saw is usually used nowadays and the table set to cut the sloping side at the required angle. Cleaning up after making the second cut (facing the jacks) is easier if the bridge is temporarily supported against the part of the board from which it was separated by the first cut. A convenient temporary fixing can be made by gluing a number of small patches of scrap soundboard wood under the bridge and under part of the board, with the grain running across the cut which separates them.

To guide the placing of the bridge pins, Keene seems to have made a series of fine knife lines across the sloping top surface of the bridge and parallel to the back of the instrument. These are shown on the full-sized drawing. Most of these lines run between a close pair of bridge pins. There are, however, 11 extra lines which may have had a different purpose or may have been due to a false start. It is probably safer nowadays to copy the bridge-pin positions from the full-sized drawing (but do *not* copy the nut pin positions).

The holes for the bridge pins can be made with a twist drill, but they are very conveniently bored with an awl specially made from a short piece of piano wire mounted in a pin vice. The piano wire is ground to a chisel edge and the awl is started by pressing it into the bridge with its edge at right angles to the grain before twisting it to and fro. If you are copying Keene in having two sizes of bridge pins, you will need two sizes of awl. The awl works well on sloping surfaces, which are awkward for a drill.

The best time to glue the bridge to the soundboard is after the bridge-pin holes have been made, but before the pins are fitted. Keene marked all round the bridge on the soundboard with a scriber and then roughened the underside of the bridge and the surface of the soundboard within the scribed line by removing tiny chips in a random pattern. These marks can be seen in photographs 1 and 9.

The soundboard is the most easily damaged part of the instrument, and may need to be repaired at some time in the future. It is best, therefore, if a water-soluble glue is used for gluing on the bridge and bars; for gluing the soundboard to the liners, and the mouldings and hitchrails to the soundboard. These parts can then be taken apart without damaging them.

Before gluing on the bridge, the soundboard should be in equilibrium with slightly drier air than it will normally meet. (A board as thin as this reaches equilibrium in a few hours.) Then its normal condition in the instrument is one of slight compression. Keene used 10 small tacks to reinforce the joint between the soundboard and the bridge, and probably put them in after the glue was dry. If the soundboard is held up to the light the position of the edges of the bridge can be seen from underneath and the tacks can be placed. Alternatively 10 holes could have been made from above within the scribed line before the bridge was glued on, and these holes used to position the tacks from underneath.

It is easier to knock in the bridge pins before the bars are glued to the underside of the soundboard. The tops of Keene's pins were neatly levelled with a file. These pins can be made from brass wire if the right combination of diameter and length is not available. The bars should be glued into place after the bridge pins have been fitted and when the soundboard has been brought back into equilibrium with air of the same humidity that was chosen when the bridge was glued on. Bringing the soundboard into equilibrium amounts to shrinking it across the grain until it is a suitable width to be fixed by the bars. Another way of controlling the width is to mark an arbitrary dimension across the grain under the soundboard in several places and warm the board uniformly (warm air is a convenient method) until it has shrunk by a standard ratio (e.g. 1 in 150).

The liner must be recessed under the ends of the bars. While the soundboard is being glued in, enough temporary strips, about 12×12 mm in section, will be needed to hold it down all round its edge, including the edge adjoining the jack guide. These strips should be held down, while the glue dries, by nails which can be easily pulled out, and to save time during the gluing process, these nails should have been knocked in, but left so that they just do not pierce the lower surface. Keene's nails were about 100 mm apart. If animal glue is used, it should be very weak and free flowing. This is partly because the glue is bound to cool and thicken somewhat during the time taken to place the soundboard and nail down the temporary strips, and partly because a soundboard as thin as this one can be adequately held by a bond of moderate strength. The bond between the soundboard and the bridge, on the other hand, needs considerable strength because the tension of the strings tends to pull the joint apart, particularly in the treble.

The arrangements for gluing in the soundboard need to be well prepared so that there is no unnecessary delay between applying the glue and nailing down the temporary strips. It is better if two people, each with a glue brush and a hammer, can share the task. The jack guide should be masked so that the glue can be spread quickly without worrying about any which overlaps the guide. The liners should be made fairly hot, for instance by using two electric radiant strip heaters which can be moved from one part to another and back again. As soon as the source of heat is withdrawn, the hot thin glue should be applied quickly and liberally to the liners, the soundboard positioned tightly against the jack guide with small gaps along the other edges, and the temporary strips nailed down firmly. Two people should complete this process, from the withdrawal of the heaters to the nailing of the strips in less than a minute.

An alternative method of heating the liners makes use of burning shavings from hand-planing operations (not sawdust or chips from chiselling). The shavings are gathered to form a narrow band on the table, following the shape of the liners when the case is upside-down. There should be sufficient shavings to burn for about half a minute. The whole band is then ignited and the spinet case inverted so that the liners are directly above the flames all the way round. Just before the flames die down the case is turned the right way up and hot glue spread on the hot liners as described above. There tends to be some soot and slight charring in places, but the liners will not be burned by such a brief exposure. It is a wise precaution to have a bucket of sand, a can of water or a fire extinguisher in case of emergencies. The masking of the jack guide needs to resist the flames, perhaps by being slightly damp. The pearwood veneer will later cover any soot or marks of charring on the inside of the case walls. Keene does not seem to have used this method, although other makers did, since there is no trace of soot on the liners, but he may have turned the case on its back and warmed the inside in front of a wide fire.

When the glue between the soundboard and the liners is dry the temporary strips are removed and the nail holes which will show, i.e. those near the jack guide, are plugged with small splints of wood. Then the pearwood veneer is glued round the inside of the case. The way in which the joints of Keene's veneer overlap in the corners of the case is shown on the full-sized plan, and indicates that he began by fitting the veneer inside the tail. When the glue between the veneer and the case is dry the top surface of all the case walls should be planed level and covered with walnut crossbanding about 3 mm thick. Crossbanding was probably used because it can be jointed as many times as necessary without the joints being noticeable. Then the soundboard mouldings and hitchrails can be glued down. Keene nailed these down, leaving the nails in place. The hitchrail for the bentside was kerfed in 13 places to make it easy to bend. He also glued on and nailed the baseboard mouldings; the profile of these is shown on the full-sized drawing.

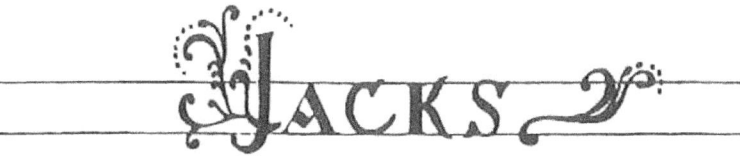

Jacks

TYPICAL jacks made during the seventeenth century and early part of the eighteenth have construction marks on the front face like those shown in figure 16. These were intended to help someone working on one jack at a time and using tools which allowed him to see the marks as he cut and drilled. As jacks made in London in the late eighteenth century have no construction lines on their faces, they must have been made using jigs, and this would have facilitated the large-scale production achieved by workshops like those of Shudi and Kirkman. The earlier method of jack making will be described here, since it is simple and uses few special tools. Makers nowadays who wish to make more than about a thousand jacks will be able to devise methods which will speed production once the time has been spent on making the jigs. As always, elaboration is easier than simplification.

Jacks are made by preparing blocks of pearwood as shown in figure 13 so that each time a slice is sawn off the block, a strip is produced which only needs planing to thickness for it to be able to move up and down in the register slots. Pearwood is usually chosen (though the Italians used other fruitwoods and Ruckers used beech) because it is hard, is available in fairly large pieces, and planes to a very smooth finish. It will help the planing of the faces if the grain is chosen, as shown in figure 13, to run at about 5° to the edge of the block. Grain sometimes varies in direction within a block, but if you start with a small angle, you are less likely to meet any grain which cannot be planed in the chosen direction. The jack blanks should be stacked and planed in the order that they were cut from the block, so that each jack as it is planed gives a warning of what imperfections to expect when planing the next. The simplest way to keep the blanks in the order in which they were cut is to make a diagonal pencil line across the block, as shown in figure 13, similar to Keene's own diagonal line across the keys shown in figure 7.

Spinet and virginal jacks often have lead weights to make them weigh as much as normal harpsichord jacks. The easiest way of forming these weights is to drill a deep blind hole in each jack block and fill it with molten lead. The jack block can then be sawn and the blanks planed as if they were only wood. It is advisable to tap the lead on each side of the blank with a ball-faced hammer to tighten it; any dents in the lead surface will disappear when the jack is planed. Lead and the fumes of lead are poisonous, so care is needed. Both the lead and the hole must be dry, or there might be a small explosion due to the formation of steam, so it is a wise precaution to wear goggles.

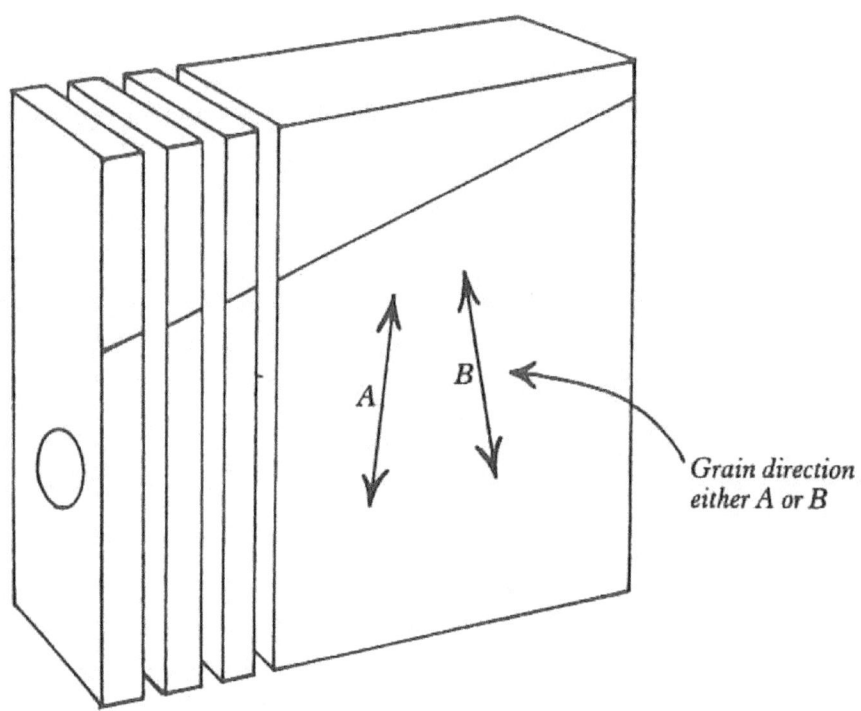

Fig. 13 Jack blanks cut from a prepared block

Figure 14 shows an old teaspoon with the tip bent to form a pouring lip, so that it is rather like a grapefruit spoon. A small teaspoon will fill a hole 7 mm in diameter by about 70 mm deep. Hold the spoon in a fold of cloth and melt a few small pieces of lead in it over a gas flame. Then the surface of the molten lead is skimmed to remove any dross, the tip of the spoon is placed against the hole in the jack block and the lead poured in slowly. As shown in figure 14, the jack block should be held at an angle of about 20° to the horizontal. The lead should be only a little above melting point. If this method is followed, the lead flows from the spoon to the hole until the hole is full. Then the block can be raised gradually and the spoon withdrawn.

The jack blanks sawn from the block are placed in a groove as shown in figure 15 and planed until the surface is level with the top of the groove. The blank is then equal in thickness to the depth of the groove, which can be adjusted by taking shavings off or by gluing strips of paper on the bottom. The groove can be cut with a plough or combination plane or

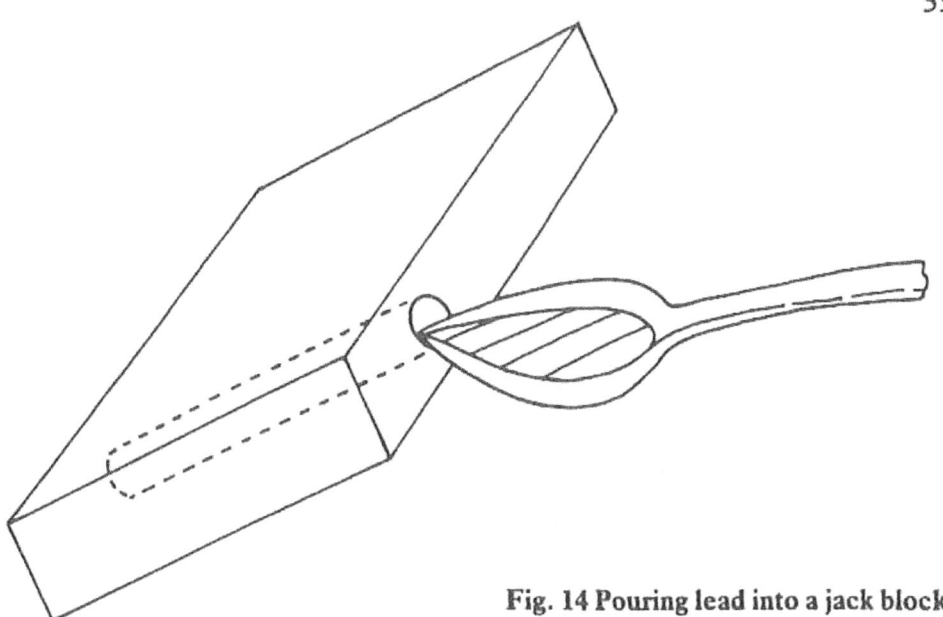

Fig. 14 Pouring lead into a jack block

built up by gluing strips onto a block. It is an advantage to have a slightly shallower groove alongside the first into which the blank can be inverted so that the second side can be planed. The first groove can be uniform in depth, but the second groove determines the exact thickness of the jack at each point, and if the jack is to be tapered, as most old jacks are, the groove needs to be deeper at the end intended for the top of the jack. The purpose of tapering the jacks is to make them easier to get in and out of the jack slots, and Keene's nameboard was tapered for the same reason.

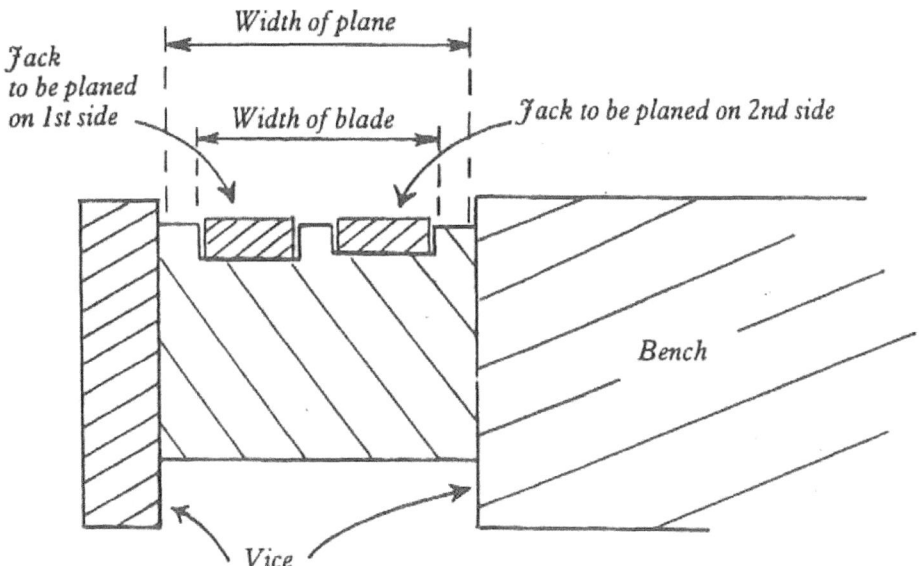

Fig. 15 Thicknessing of jacks

The jack slots, however, are not tapered, probably because the fit of the jack at the bottom of the slot has hardly any effect on the plucking of the string.

The side-by-side grooves can be used together, one jack having its front face planed while the other is being finished to thickness. The plane can usually be set to reduce the blanks to the required thicknesses in about five or six strokes. This process is quite rapid, therefore, and great uniformity can be achieved with care. Usually, however, the problem is to make a jack fit a particular slot in the jack guide. If the second groove is set to make jacks which fit the wider slots, the jacks for the narrower slots can be produced by laying one or two loose strips of paper under the jack in the second groove. Jacks which have a clearance in the thickness of 0.2 mm work well and do not stick in damp weather. The side clearance can be 0.4 mm or more. The jacks should be numbered as they are removed from the slots.

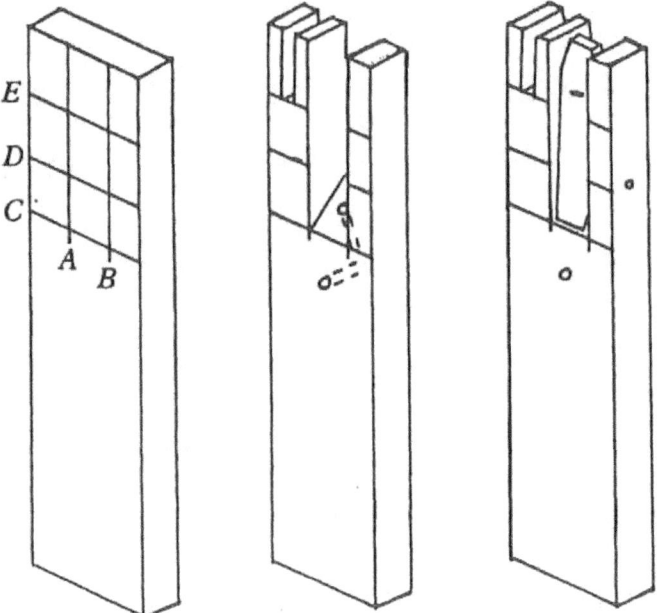

Fig. 16 Stages in making a jack

Figure 16 shows the usual way to mark out jacks to be finished by eye using simple hand tools. Diderot's *Encyclopedie* published between 1751 and 1758 actually illustrates a *Trace-sauteraux* for marking out jacks (see Hubbard, pl. 32, fig. 14) but an ordinary mortice gauge can be used. To saw down the sides of all the tongue slots is somewhat time consuming (perhaps an hour for a set of jacks) and it is worth setting up a carbide-tipped circular saw if one is available, especially if it is wobbled slightly to cut a slot 4.5 mm wide. But hand sawing is quite convenient if a dovetail saw is used with the jack horizontal and overhanging the back of a block, the saw blade being held parallel to the slope at the bottom of the tongue slot. The piece between the two cuts can be removed with a chisel, the cut being made slightly above line c. After this chisel cut has removed most of the waste, the final cut can be made on line c with the slope shown on the twice-full-sized detail on the drawing. The two sawn sides can be smoothed with a file if the saw has not left them smooth enough. The sawcut for the damper should be made with a fairly coarse saw, as some roughness in the kerf helps to grip the cloth.

The two holes near the bottom of the tongue slot for the bristle spring need to be about 0.6 mm diameter to suit hog bristles that are between 0.4 and 0.5 mm thick. Many eighteenth-century harpsichords still have their original bristle springs in working order, showing that this is a very reliable material. These holes are easily drilled with a piece of piano wire held in a pin vice, the end of the wire being sharp enough if it is cut with nippers – not shears. The pin vice is twisted between the fingers and the wire gradually worked into the jack. The position and angle of the lower hole are not critical, as its purpose is to prevent the bristle from moving, but allow it to be changed without difficulty. The position and angle of the upper hole are critical, and while it is possible, with care, to drill it freehand it is easy enough to construct a drilling jig to ensure uniformity. A suitable jig is shown in figure 17. It is difficult to drill the guide hole in the jig so that it passes through the block at the correct angle using a wire as the drill, but if the hole is made so that it runs in approximately the

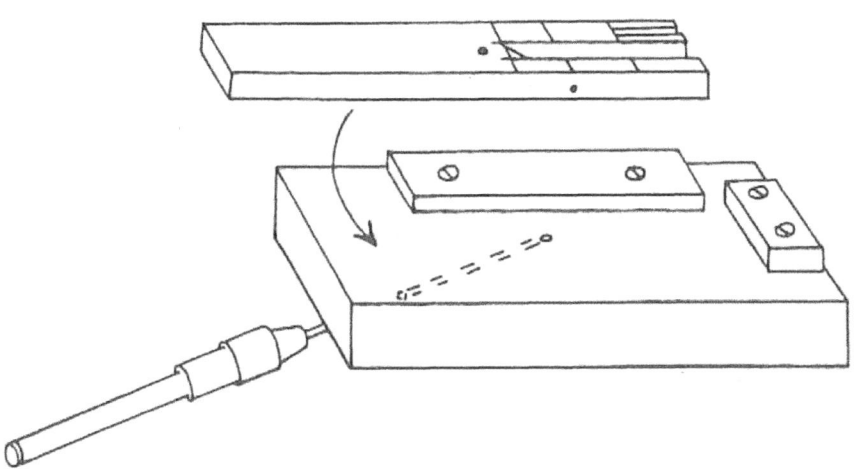

Fig. 17 Drilling the oblique bristle hole

right direction, the angle that the surface makes with the hole can be adjusted by using a plane to slope the upper surface of the block. Two pieces of wood are then attached to the top surface to locate each jack while the bristle hole is being drilled. The wire can be rotated by an electric drill if the number of jacks to be made is thought to justify it. The advantages of drilling with a wire are: that it does not enlarge the guide hole by cutting the sides, as an ordinary twist drill would do, and it does not clog with wood dust. The wood dust is simply compressed into the sides of the drilled hole. The small patch of white leather shown on the double-sized drawing of the jack is a usual refinement on English eighteenth-century jacks and makes the action a little quieter. All the jacks of the Keene and Brackley spinet are lost, so the drawing shows jacks from a spinet by Keene c. 1680 in the Royal College of Music, London.

The tongues can be made from strips of holly with a section of 33 × 2.8 mm cut with the grain running across the 33 mm width. Three or four strips will be needed to make sufficient tongues for one spinet, because the lengths of the strips must total about 320 mm. The profile given on the drawing can be worked with a chisel on each strip, guided by the four construction lines indicated in figure 18. The V-shaped nick at the back of each tongue is usual on English jacks. It was copied from jacks made by the Ruckers family, and was probably intended to help position a punch held in the hand and tapped with a hammer.

The punch is shown in figure 18. It can be made from about 70 mm of gauge 20 piano wire (1.15 mm diameter) held in a pin vice and flattened (cold) with a hammer and anvil until a length of about 10 mm at one end has become about 1.8 mm wide and 0.6 mm thick. A few millimeters should be clipped off the end in case it is cracked, and the tip should then be rubbed on a coarse sharpening stone to taper both flat sides symmetrically to a chisel edge. The punch should then be moved in the pin vice so that it is held very tightly with about 6 mm protruding.

Before the plectrum hole is punched, the front edge of the tongue strip should be shot with a plane and marked with gauge lines to indicate the finished width. The punch can then be positioned by eye half-way across the marked width and tapped with a light hammer to drive it through the tongue strip and into a hardwood backing piece, so that the hole slopes upwards at about 5°. The punch can be withdrawn easily with a side-to-side movement. The relief for the bristle is also shown in figure 18. It is cut by eye with two strokes of a chisel or one stroke of an engraver's burin so that it is half-way across the marked width of the tongue. Then the tongue is sawn from the strip and the process repeated for the next tongue. To complete each tongue, shoot its second side with a plane and round both sides a little with a chisel at top and bottom as shown in the full-sized drawing. The top reliefs are important, since the damper cloth tends to deform the damper slot slightly, bending one side towards the tongue.

Each finished tongue is paired off with a finished body, and the two pieces held together so that the tongue is in the correct rest position shown in figure 16 and in the full-sized drawing. As explained below, the front face of the tongue is not vertical, but slopes backwards at an angle of about 3°, the foot of the tongue being flush with the front of the body and the back of the quill flush with the back of the body. The pivot hole is then bored level with line D which is marked on the jack face, through the narrow side of the fork, through the tongue and a little way into the wider side of the fork. This hole should be a push fit on the axle, (a dressmaker's brass pin of about 0.6 mm diameter is ideal, otherwise a piece of brass wire), but the hole in the tongue should be redrilled to enlarge it to give a generous clearance over the axle. The tongue is also given a generous clearance in the fork – 0.2 mm is about right. A precision metal-worker will perhaps think this excessive, but old jacks that are made like this are very reliable. The tongue should move freely at this stage, and if it does not, the pin can still be withdrawn easily. If the tongue moves freely, a bristle can be pushed up the inclined hole to lie along the V-shaped relief. The tongue should then remain in position with the jack held horizontally face upwards, but move when blown

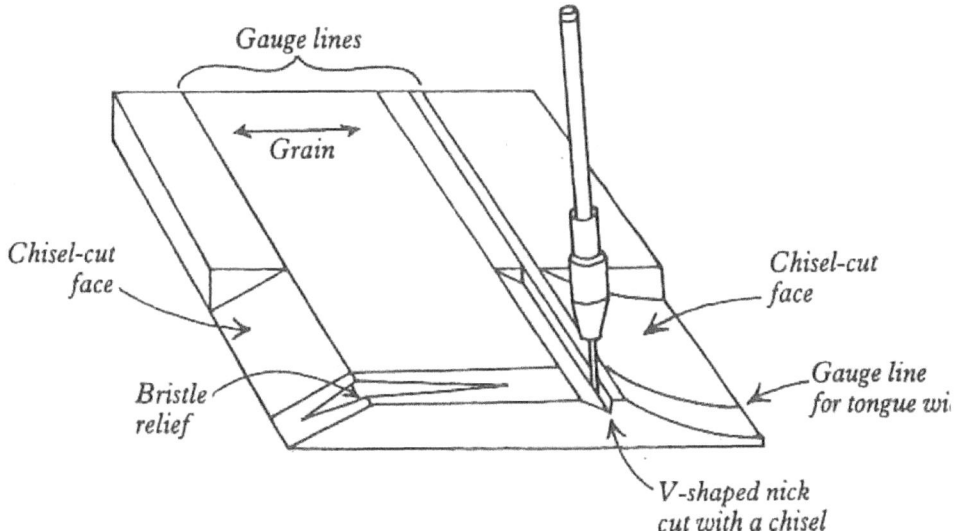

Fig. 18 Punching the plectrum holes in the tongue strip

downwards. If the bristle is satisfactory, the lower end is looped into the transverse hole in the jack, pulled through and cut off flush with the front of the jack. Bristles between 0.4 mm and 0.5 mm diameter are of suitable strength, but the diameter varies along the bristle, gradually decreasing away from the pig and usually ending in a number of separate wisps which must be cut off. A good bristle will serve two or three jacks. After cutting off the bristle, the axle can be clipped close to the side of the jack and filed flush.

Tongues are hardly ever troublesome, but if one needs to be withdrawn after the axle has been cut off, the axle can be cut through with a ground-down hacksaw blade worked between the tongue and the narrow side of the forked part of the jack. The tongue can then be twisted to remove both it and part of the axle, while the rest of the axle can be pushed into the tongue slot.

The slight backward slope of the tongue in its rest position, which was mentioned above, is usual in English jacks. Presumably, the intention was to gain the maximum length of quill and at the same time keep the tongue entirely within the body of the jack when it was at rest. If the tongue had been placed vertically and flush with the front of the jack body, the quill would have been about 1.2 mm shorter. The sloped tongue position also helps to tilt the quill. A quill works best if it is tilted upwards by about 8° relative to the front of the jack body, mostly because the bristle can then be slightly stronger without causing the quill to hang on the string. The angle of tilt of the quill slot relative to the front of the tongue should thus be about 5°.

Wooden jacks can be bought, though not precisely to this elegant early English design. In these pages I have tried to show that jack making is not difficult and does not need many special tools.

Stringing and Quilling

THE treble string lengths of a keyboard instrument are characterised by its so-called 'scale', which is the nominal length between nut and bridge of the string sounding c^2. If the scale is perfectly adhered to, the string lengths of all the treble strings will vary inversely as the frequency of the notes they sound, so that the length of c^2 is doubled for c^1 and halved for c^3. This applies only in the treble, since the bass strings are always shortened in order to fit them into a manageable size of case. Usually the lengths of the highest strings and those in the middle of the compass are made slightly shorter than the theoretical scale. This is done for two reasons. Firstly, it is difficult to make the lengths of the short strings accurate in the top octave, so they are usually made slightly shorter than the theoretical length to ensure that errors do not make them too long. Strings that are too long need to be held at a greater tension, and this can cause them to break. Secondly, the string lengths are sometimes reduced in the middle of the compass to allow for the tendency of thicker strings to have a slightly lower tensile strength than those that are thinner.

In a spinet or virginal there is another effect modifying the string lengths. The placing of strings in pairs shortens all the strings which lie to the right of their jacks compared with the lengths they would have had if the strings had been equally spaced. This shortening is usually about 4%, making their lengths the same as if they had been calculated from a c^2 string that was 4% shorter. Strings which lie to the left of their jacks must have a scale that gives a suitable safety factor between their actual pitch and the pitch at which they would break. This gives a safety factor to the strings which lie to the right of their jacks which is 4% greater, with the disadvantage that they do not sound quite so true.

If the string lengths of an old instrument are measured it is often difficult to be sure which departures from an exact scale are deliberate and which are accidental. Keene has chosen string lengths which conform fairly accurately to a scale of 267 mm between notes e and c^3. This scale was probably chosen because it was 10½ inches on Keene's rule. The inaccuracies in this part of the compass seem to be random, including lengths 3% reduced near note d and 1% increased at f♯ and f♯². Above c^3, the reductions of length appear to be deliberate, reaching 8% at e^3. Below e the string lengths are limited by the case dimensions and bridge design, the string lengths of c, C and GG being respectively 96%, 66% and 52% of those necessary to maintain the treble scale. This represents a fairly generous compromise which gives excellent sound at c, good sound at C and passable sound at GG. A longer case would have made the bass notes sound better and a shorter case would have made them sound worse.

While you can position the nut satisfactorily by following the full-sized drawing, it is better to measure string lengths. The positions of the bridge pins and the jacks have already been fixed, and some deviations from the drawing are likely to have occurred. It is therefore advantageous to follow the second rule mentioned in the Introduction and to measure some chosen string lengths from the actual bridge pins and past the actual jacks in a position which will give the quills a good length. I suggest that you keep the nut straight, but position it so that the e string measures 848 mm and the e^2 string measures 212 mm. If the length of the e^1 string is measured to this nut position it should be about 424 mm. A small deviation from this figure will not matter, but if it is more than 428 mm, the nut should be moved towards the bridge to reduce it to 424 mm. If the length of the e^3 string is then checked, it should measure about 98 mm. If it is more than about 104 mm the nut should be moved a little to reduce the length. A nut position established by this method will give the best possible string lengths and allow for any variations of bridge and jack positions which have occurred. When the nut position is considered satisfactory a straight line should be scribed on the wrestplank either side of the nut, as Keene did.

The original nut has seven nails in the long part and two in the short bass end set along a scribed line at the ridge. Holes for these nails must be drilled through the nut, but the nails can find their own way into the wrestplank. The nails should be driven nearly through the nut, the two jointing surfaces heated, then hot glue applied to the underside of the nut and the joint rubbed to and fro, leaving it between the scribed lines. Finally the nails are driven home to secure the joint.

Keene scribed another line along the nut 2.7 mm from the ridge to mark where the nut pins were to go. This implies that he had a separate method for locating them laterally along the line, probably something like the method shown in figure 19. This employs a loop of wire and a pair of sharp points made from bridge pins and set 4.5 mm apart in a piece of hardwood. The loop of wire is hitched over one of the hitchpins and drawn forward past the bridge pins for notes c♯³ and d³ and touching the pair of points. The pair of points is then positioned over the scribed line on the nut and moved along the nut until the two sides of the loop are half-way between the jacks for c♯³ and d³. Then the points are pressed into the nut on the scribed line making two marks where the two nut pins must go. The loop is then taken past the bridge pins for b² and c³, the wires positioned midway between the jacks for b² and c³ and another pair of nut-pin marks made. When all the nut pins have been marked in this way, the nut-pin holes should be made, like the bridge-pin holes, with a special awl or a twist drill, and the nut pins inserted.

Tuning pins of the kind used by Keene can easily be made by sawing mild steel rod or nails of 4.4 mm diameter into 46 mm lengths. The rod is rotated in a lathe or drill, while one end is filed to the taper shown on the full-sized drawing, leaving the taper with a fairly accurate profile but with a slightly rough finish. At the same time the surface of the rod should be scratched with a file at the part where the wire will be wound on, because otherwise the wire does not grip easily. Keene would not have had this problem; his rod would have been rough enough because of the way it was made. The other end is flattened a little using a hammer and anvil. There is no harm in using modern 5 mm square-headed zither pins which have a hole for the wire, and a parallel shank with a lightly engraved spiral; but traditional pins are not difficult to wind with the kind of wire used on spinets and the taper enables you to adjust the grip to give easy but precise tuning. It would be difficult to persuade violinists to abandon their tapered tuning pegs.

Keene's tuning-pin positions are not very regular and there seems to be no obvious reason behind their irregularity, which has the effect of

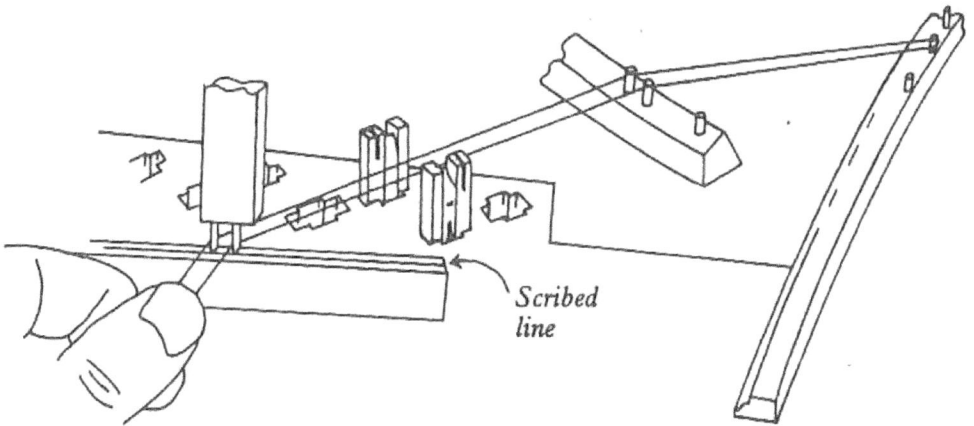

Fig. 19 Marking the nut pin positions

increasing the side-draught between notes f and b¹ to between 15° and 20°, whereas it is only 10° at c♯³. If you decide to maintain 10° over the whole range (and this will be found to be sufficient) the easiest way of marking the tuning-pin holes is with an ordinary adjustable bevel used as shown in figure 20. The two lines along which the tuning pins above G are placed, are parallel to the main part of the nut and are 21 mm and 34 mm from its front edge. For each tuning pin position, the bevel is lined up with the nut pin, a tuning pin is placed on the appropriate line and touching the bevel, and the pin tapped with a hammer to mark the wrestplank. If, on the other hand, you decide to copy Keene's variable side-draft angles, you can copy the tuning pin positions from the drawing. The tapered pins can be inserted into an ordinary parallel-sided hole drilled in the wrestplank, or a special tapered drill can be made by grinding the end like a tuning pin. The drill should be about 0.2 mm smaller than the diameter of the tuning pin and the hole should be drilled deep enough to leave a small vacant space below the pin when this is in place. You should drill the wrestplank, canting the drill so that it is at right angles to the strings, which slope towards the wrestplank after they have passed over the nut.

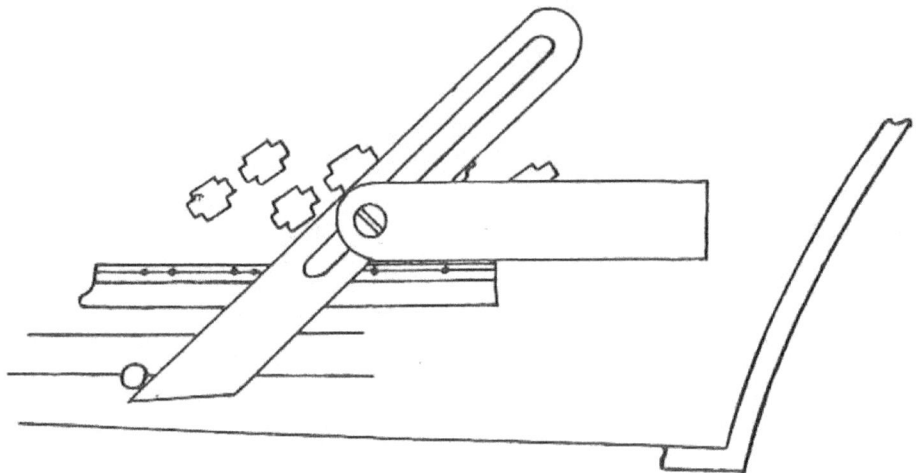

Fig. 20 Marking the tuning pin positions

Figure 21 shows how the wire is unwound from a reel and a loop is made at the end to attach the string to a hitch pin. Many tuning keys have survived from the eighteenth century, and most have a hook for winding loops, but a substitute can be made by screwing a small hook into a short length of dowel. The wire from the reel is passed over the hook and held in the left hand near its end. The right hand, holding the dowel or tuning key, then rotates the hook and winds a spiral, the wire being kept taut by the restraint mounted next to the reel and by pulling with the hands. Twisting the hook has the effect of twisting the end held in the left hand and also the wire coming from the reel. The distance between reel and loop needs therefore to be sufficient for the wire to receive about 8 complete turns without passing its elastic limit. If soft brass is used for the lowest notes, the distance may need to be 3 m. Loops in thick wire need to be wound under greater tension than those in thin wire, which may involve tightening the restraint screws. It is better to start stringing at the top note so that you are used to handling thin strings before having to deal with thicker ones.

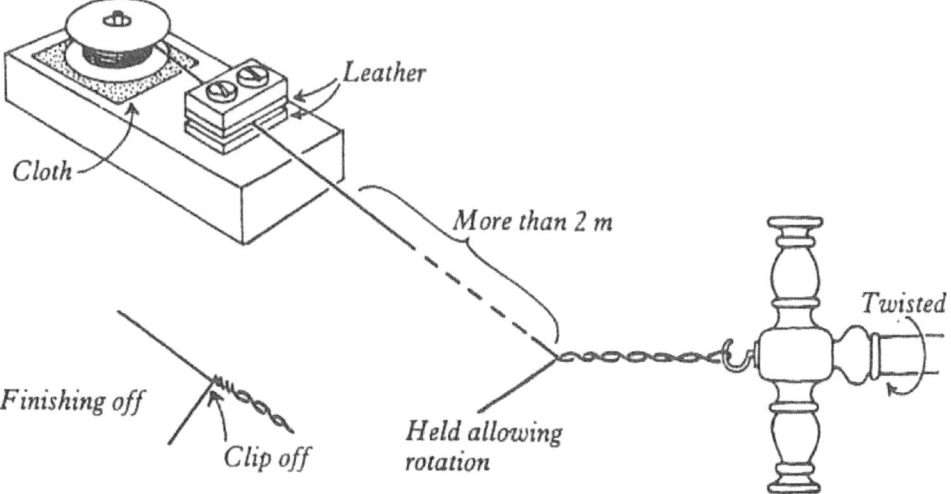

Fig. 21 Winding loops

Figure 22 shows how the wire is wound on the tuning pin. All the pins are worked into their holes with the tuning key, leaving their tops level with each other. They are then marked at the point where the winding needs to start, so that the wires between the nut and the various tuning pins have a uniform slope and a tidy appearance. Each pin is withdrawn with the tuning key as it is required. The previously wound loop is placed over the appropriate hitch pin, the string taken past the corresponding bridge pin and held so that it passes above the corresponding tuning pin hole. For the thinnest strings, a kink is made in the wire at a point about 210 mm past the hole. This allows sufficient wire to wrap round the tuning pin about fourteen times. Then the wire is cut at about 70 mm past the kink and the winding started as shown in figure 22, placing the kink on the mark. Using both hands, the spiral must be held firmly against the tuning pin until the wire has been wound tightly over the spiral several times. The string must be kept taut while you are holding the pin and following the procedure shown in figure 22. When you are ready to press the tuning pin into its hole, the right hand holds the pin while the left hand pulls the string aside a little to the left, near the point where it passes over the row of jacks. The left hand continues to keep the string taut while the right hand leaves the pin wedged into the top of its hole, picks up the tuning key and twists the tuning pin to and fro while pressing it home. The left hand then guides the string round the appropriate pin on the nut, the right hand tightens the string with the tuning key and the left hand can then be withdrawn. If you wish the thicker wires to form windings on tuning pins of similar appearance to those of the thinner wires, the number of turns should be reduced for each increase in thickness, so that it varies from fourteen in the treble to about seven in the bass. This involves a gradual reduction in the length of wire allowed between the tuning pin hole and the kink. It is useful to have these lengths marked with the corresponding gauges on a measuring stick which can be held against the string.

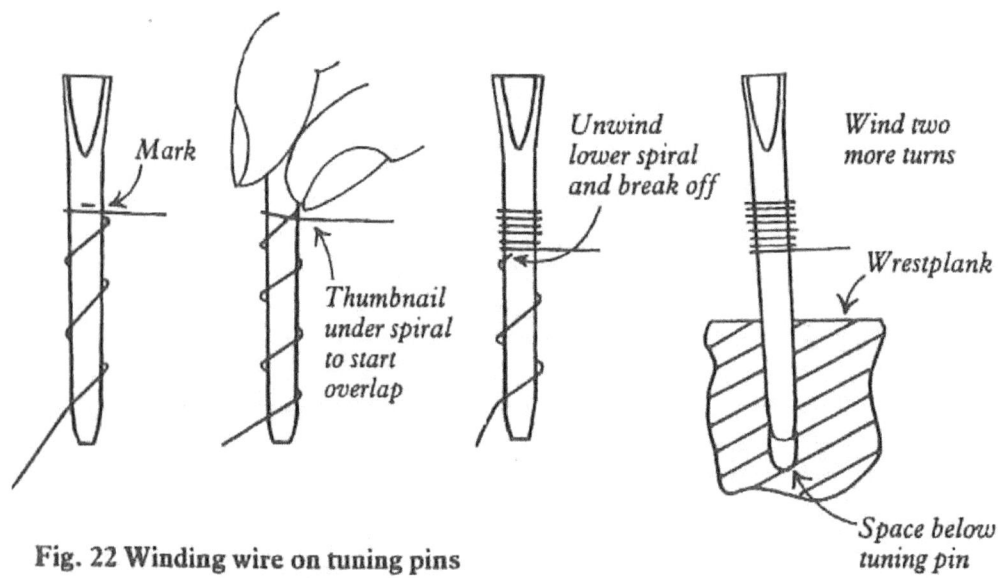

Fig. 22 Winding wire on tuning pins

Keene did not record the gauge numbers of his strings, and so my recommendations on the full-sized drawing are based on the gauges marked on an anonymous spinet dated 1708 in the Royal College of Music, London. These gauges were probably added c. 1740. The positions of the transitions from one gauge to the next can be moved up or down the keyboard if it seems to improve the sound. Thinner strings sound truer because their harmonics are more nearly in tune with the fundamental, but they also limit the strength of the quills that can be used, because if plucked beyond a certain limit, thin strings will not absorb the energy of strong quills and will produce an unpleasant sound of ill-defined pitch, a condition known as 'over-plucking'.

The best quills are those of raven or vulture, especially for the thick bass strings, but crow quills are satisfactory and are more readily available, since crows are often shot by gamekeepers in the course of their work. The feathers to use are the six or eight largest flight feathers from an adult bird, each of which usually supplies three or four plectra. A single raven feather, however, will often quill twelve jacks. The best knife to use is a surgical scalpel with a no. 3 holder and a no. 11 blade. The vane is stripped off first, leaving the shaft of the feather, the tip of which will be too weak even for treble plectra. With the black part against a block of wood, as shown in figure 23, a sloping cut at about 10° to the horizontal is made towards the end, and the tip flexed to see whether it is strong enough for one of the top notes. If not, another cut is made further down. The tip of the feather is simply pushed through the

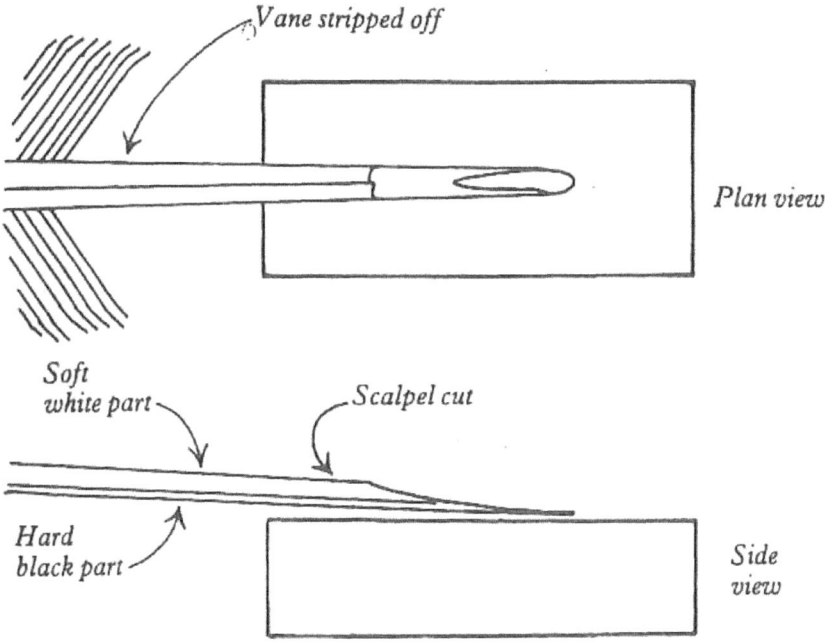

Fig. 23 Cutting a feather against a wooden block

quill slot from the back of the jack, with the black side of the feather on top, until it is firmly wedged between the top and bottom of the slot. If the sloping cut has been made at a suitable angle, the quill should protrude a little way past the string when the jack is in place. The rest of the feather is then cut with scissors against the back of the tongue. The tip of the quill is then cut off parallel with the string, either by cutting downwards onto a block of wood with the quilling knife, or by using scissors, so that the end overlaps the centre line of the string. The overlap should be about 0.6 mm on the treble strings and about 0.9 mm on bass ones. The quill should now pluck a little too strongly, so that it can be voiced later, i.e. thinned until its note matches in strength that of all the other notes in the register. Beginners usually voice too loudly, since they forget that a chord of five notes is much louder than the single note they are listening to. The keys should be easy to press, but with a definite resistance as the quill bends against the string.

The foot of the jack should be cut so that the quill lies about 1.5 mm below the string. The key raises the jack by about 9 mm, so the string is released by the quill well before the jack is stopped by the jackrail.

The Keene and Brackley spinet has the remains of a front touch which is obviously old. It is not, however, shown on the drawing because I believe that it is not original. Since there is no sign of there ever having been a back touch above the tails of the keys, it would seem that originally the jackrail provided the only means of limiting the travel of the jacks and the depression of the keys. This system is unusual in English spinets, but is found almost invariably in French instruments, where it gives a positive feel to the action and minimises action noise and wear to the balance holes of the keys. It is quite likely, therefore, that Keene thought this the best system from the players' point of view. However, it is inconvenient when one is voicing because the jackrail must be removed every time the jacks are adjusted, and replaced every time the notes are tried. The temporary front touch shown in figure 24 is easily made, and it enables notes to be played with the jackrail removed. It is possible that Keene used something of this kind when voicing in his workshop. If the front of the keyframe is lifted about 25 mm, the temporary touch can be slipped in and out without disturbing the jacks.

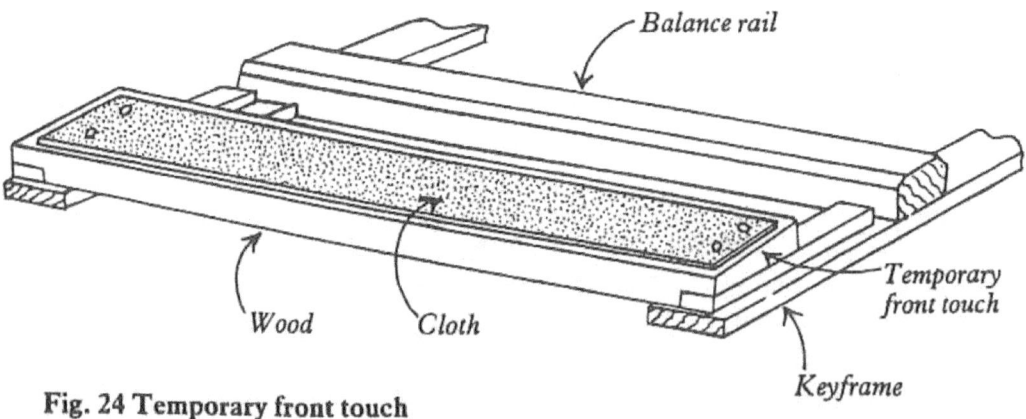

Fig. 24 Temporary front touch

The process of voicing consists in cutting thin shavings away from the underside of the quill until adjacent notes match in strength, and bass and treble stand in a suitable relationship to each other. The jack is held upside down, face forward, with the upper surface of the quill supported by a small wooden block or by the thumbnail of the left hand and cuts are made towards the tip of the quill. Shavings removed from near the jack tongue have more effect on the plucking strength than shavings removed from the tip of the quill, but the quill should taper regularly from one end to the other so that it bends in a smooth curve when pushing the string upwards. A quill that has a lot of use will become worn along the top where it touches the wire, and it will fail prematurely if the tip is too thin. Thicknesses at the tip of 0.15 mm in the treble and 0.25 mm in the bass will be found suitable. Long quills have many times the life of short quills because they are not bent so sharply. The quill must be very smooth underneath the tip, otherwise the jack will hang on the string without the tongue retracting. Olive oil is sometimes used to lubricate quills, as Adlung mentioned in his *Musica mechanica organoedi* of 1768 (see Hubbard p. 227), but in fact quills work well without oil.

Voicing should begin with a chord in the middle of the compass, e.g. f, a, c^1, f^1. These notes should not be difficult to press, nor should they sound strident when played together. Then the notes between c and c^2 should be voiced, moving up and down from c^1. The note c^2 should stand out against the chord c, e, g, c^1, and c should not be overpowered when played against the chord c^1, e^1, g^1, c^2. Then the rest of the notes can be voiced; try treble notes against bass chords, and bass notes against treble chords as well as slow chromatic scales up and down, and slow semitone trills. It will not be possible to match the sounds of strings which are plucked to the left exactly to those plucked to the right, because of the difference of scale, but there should not be sufficient difference to be noticeable when music is played.

Dampers should not be fitted until the voicing has been completed, so that the quills can be seen easily and so that nothing prevents the downward movement of the jacks. The damper in the jack shown on the full-sized drawing is cut to an approximate semicircle, and touches the string where its edge is inclined at about 45° to the horizontal. This shape is illustrated in Diderot's *Encyclopedie* (see Hubbard, pl. 40). If dampers with this contact angle are compared with the kind shaped like a square flag which touch the string with a horizontal edge, they will be found to have several advantages. They are more efficient at absorbing the string's energy; they have less tendency to curl and lose contact with the string and, like the quill when it is in contact with the string, they tend to hold the jack at the back of its slot. Dampers should be adjusted so that they have firm contact with the string but are not so low in their slots that they tend to support the jack above the key when the key has been released.

Keene scribed a bold line across the bass key-block level with the surface of the lowest key. This was probably done to record the way the instrument was originally set up, so that it could be reproduced if, for instance, the back touch cloth was changed. The position of this scribed line tallies with the bottom key as it rests on the present back touch (which is not original as was previously mentioned) and this confirms that the back touch is the correct thickness.

The original jackrail is missing from the Keene and Brackley spinet and therefore the full-sized drawing shows a reconstruction. The front and top surfaces should obviously match those of the support at the bass end, and the other features follow the pattern of contemporary spinets. The original jackrail probably had two layers of the same cloth that was used for the back touch; the cloth was probably about 1.6 mm thick when lightly compressed. The jackrail mounting pieces should be glued to the back of the case and the bentside at a height that allows the jacks to travel about 9 mm before the jackrail stops them. If the depth of the touch needs adjustment after the mounting pieces have been glued on, it may be done by using slightly thicker or thinner cloth under the jackrail.

Keene's nameboard was lettered in ink, guided by fairly bold scribed lines at the bottom and top of the small capitals. The inscription has three separate parts for each of which four impressed marks from a pointed marker can be seen. These marks stand near the ends of the scribed lines, and have obviously been made first, as a guide for positioning a ruler. The marquetry panel was cut in woods of four different colours, distinguished on the full-sized drawing by marking with dots, with a saw whose kerf measured 0.3 mm. Some of the component pieces were dipped in hot sand to darken areas meant to appear to be in shadow. The drawing shows these areas by line shading.

FURTHER READING

BLACKBURN, Graham, *The Illustrated Encyclopedia of Woodworking Handtools Instruments and Devices* John Murray, London, 1974. Alphabetical listing of tools, 238 pp, over 500 line drawings, less comprehensive than Salaman's *Dictionary of Tools* but much less expensive.

BOALCH, Donald. *Makers of the Harpsichord and Clavichord 1440-1840*. 3rd edition edited by Charles Mould; O.U.P. 1995. Alphabetical listing of over 1200 makers with biographical details and a comprehensive list of surviving instruments with their locations and owners.

GOODMAN, W.L., *The History of Woodworking Tools*, G. Bell, London, 1964. The history from Egyptian or Roman times of the axe, plane, saw, drill, bench, ruler and chisel; 208 pp. 200 figs.

HUBBARD, Frank, *Three Centuries of Harpsichord Making*, Harvard, 2nd ed. 1967 The harpsichord-maker's bible, 373 pp, 41 pls., with chapters on the various historical schools of building and old workshops, translations of old texts about harpsichords etc.

KLOP, G. C., *Harpsichord Tuning*, Garderen 1974. Obtainable from the author: Werkplaats voor Clavicimbelbouw, Garderen, Holland. A simple practical guide to tuning with details of 12 historical temperaments, 30 pp.

SALAMAN, R. A., *Dictionary of Tools used in the Woodworking and Allied Trades c. 1700–1970*, Allen & Unwin, 1975, A comprehensive alphabetical listing of tools by a collector and authority, 545 pp., 740 figs.

SCHOTT, Howard, *Playing the Harpsichord*, London, 1971. A guide to the fundamentals of harpsichord playing, including details of repertoire and basic maintenance, 223 pp., 157 musical examples.

More detailed bibliographies will be found in the above books.

SUPPLIERS

Bone: Nelson Woodworking, Jack Nelson, West Mains Road, Little Compton, Rhode Island 02837, U.S.A.

Crow feathers: James Kandik, 3618 South 18th Street, Lincoln, Nebraska 68502, USA

Jacks: Adam Swainson, Lower Pulworthy Farm, Highampton, Beaworthy, Devon, England, EX20 5LQ.

Keyfronts: Huw Saunders, 110 Milton Grove, Stoke Newington, London, England, N16 8QY.

Wire: Malcolm Rose, The Workshop, English Passage, Lewes, East Sussex, England, BN7 2AP.

Wood: North Heigham Sawmills. Paddock Street, Norwich, England NR2 41W.

Hinges: David Law, Ash House, East Street, Long Compton, Shipston-on-Stour, Warwickshire, England, CV36 SJF.

Full scale plan: Marc Vogel, Germany www.vogel-scheer.de

Second-hand furniture can often he a useful source of timber, particularly cupboards, beds and wardrobes. Solid furniture of no rarity value should be chosen and can often he found at auctions.

PHOTOGRAPHS

The following black and white photographs were taken by Peter Barnes before restoration of the spinet.

1. Treble end of wrestplank, sound board and (detached) bridge.
2. Inside of bentside from the back (sound board removed).
3. Back of keyboard rack and plan view of a2, E and BB keys.
4. Front of keyboard rack and detail of six keyfroms.
5. Nameboard and keyboard (keys b 2 - e3 separated).
6. Lid hinges and view of keyboard from treble end.
7. View of keys from underneath. showing key carving.
8. View from underneath of sound board, sound bars and bridges.

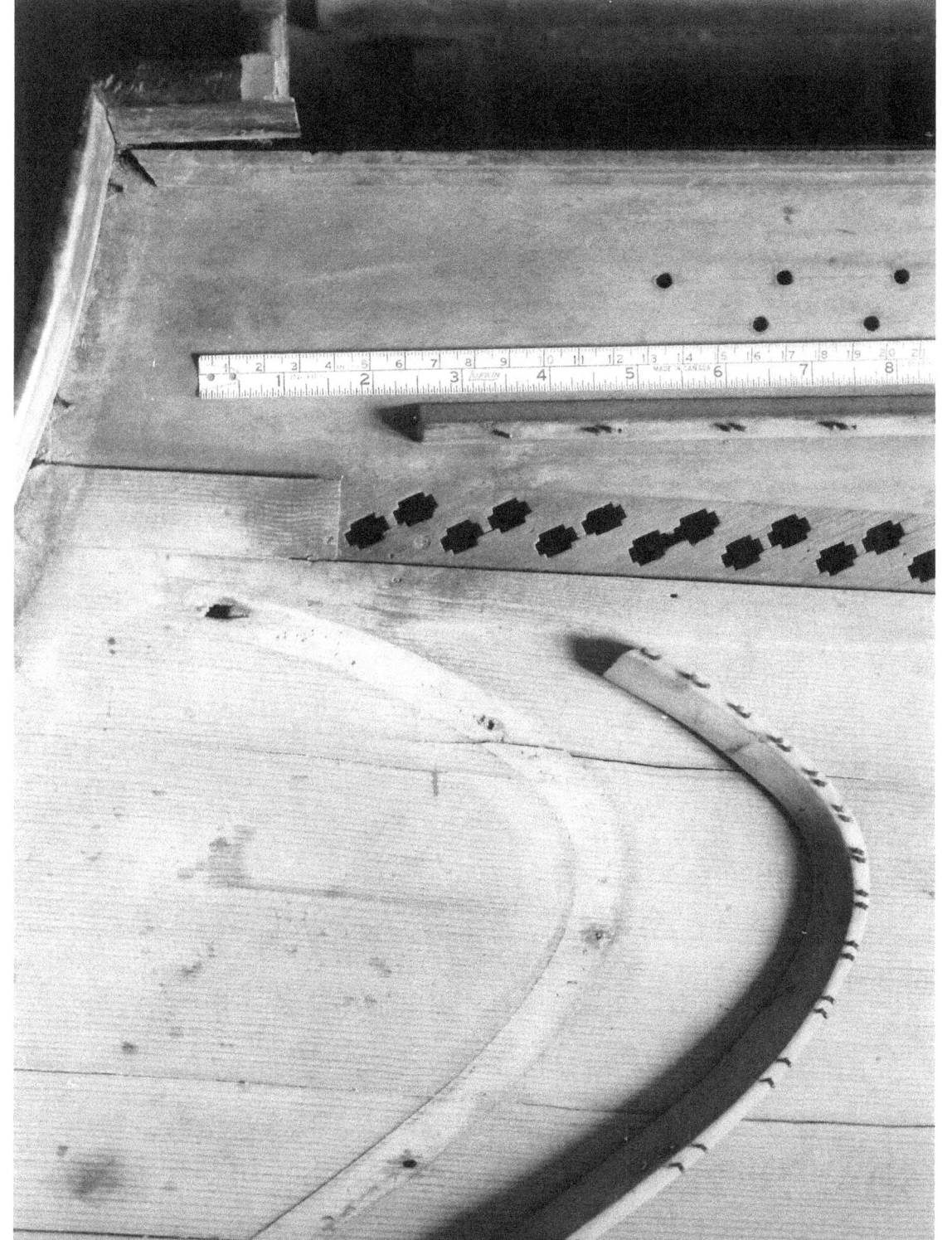

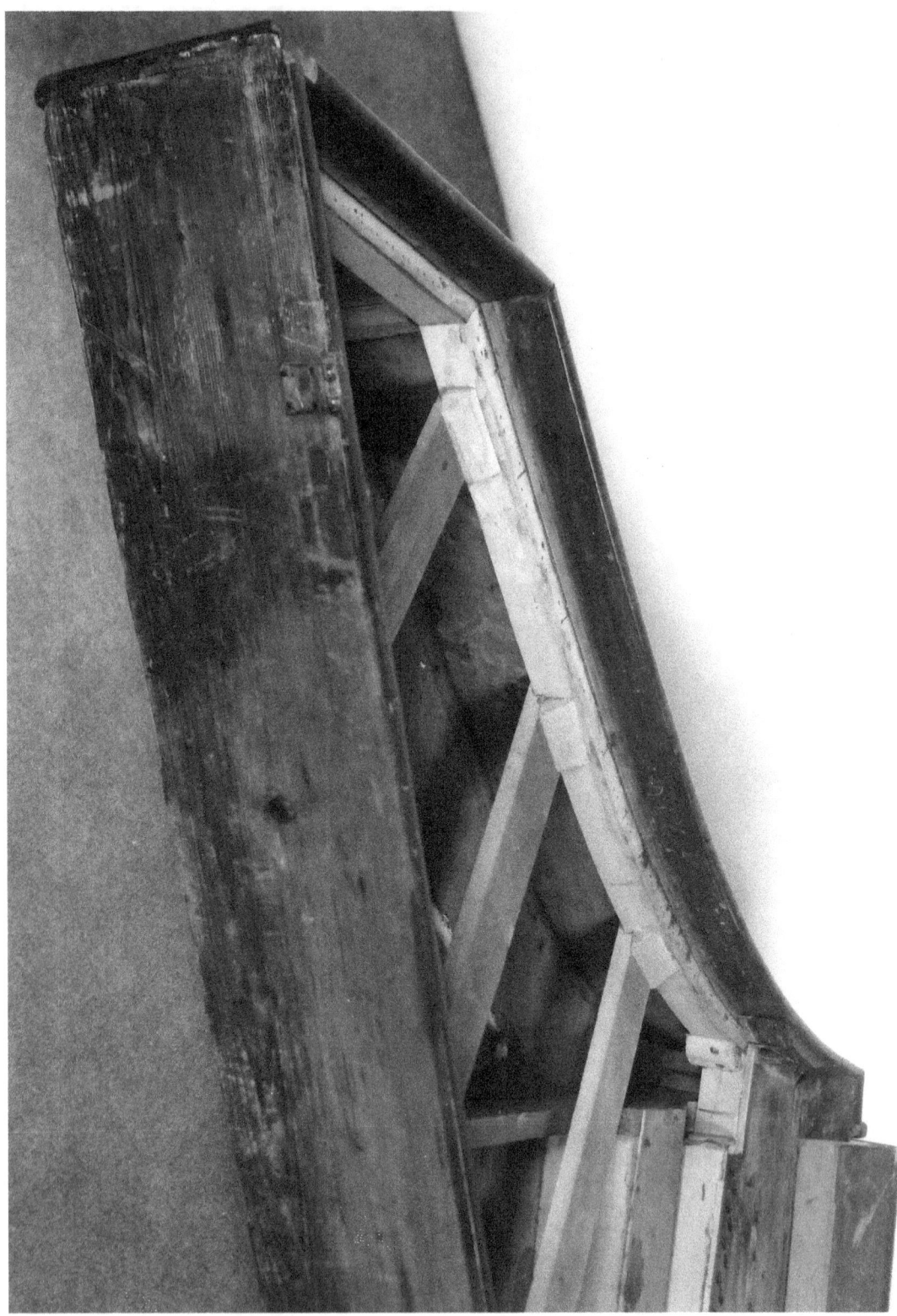

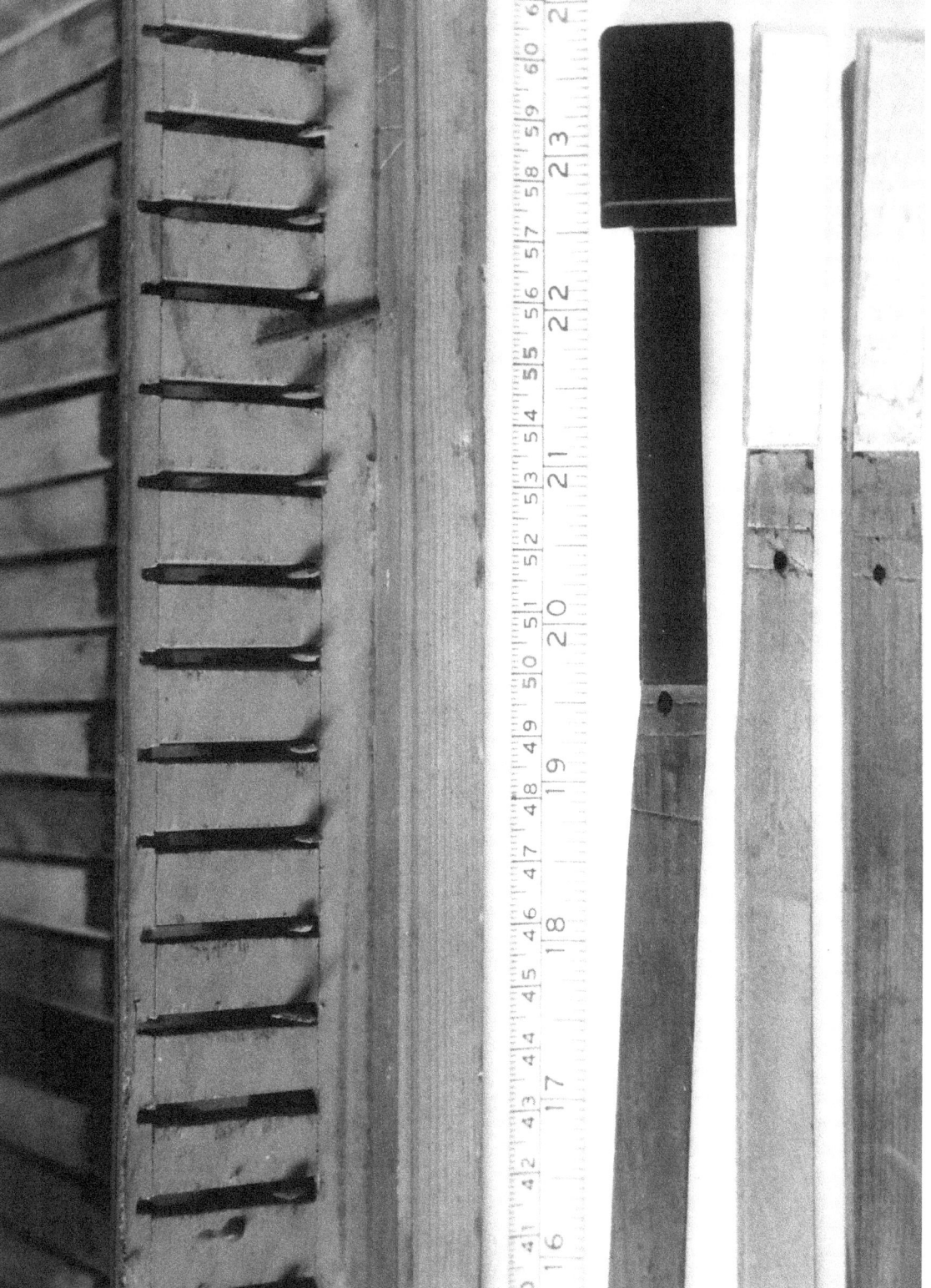

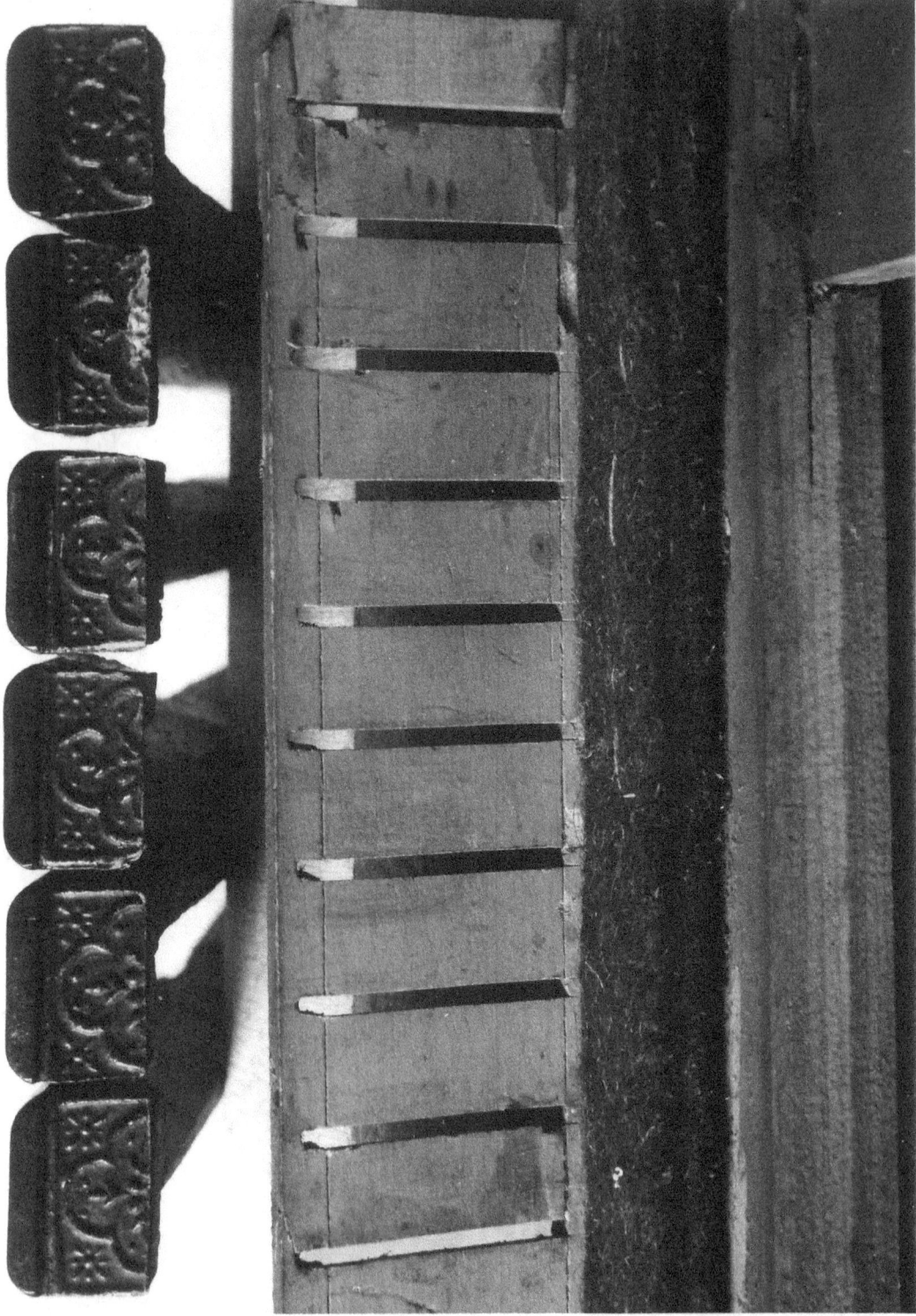

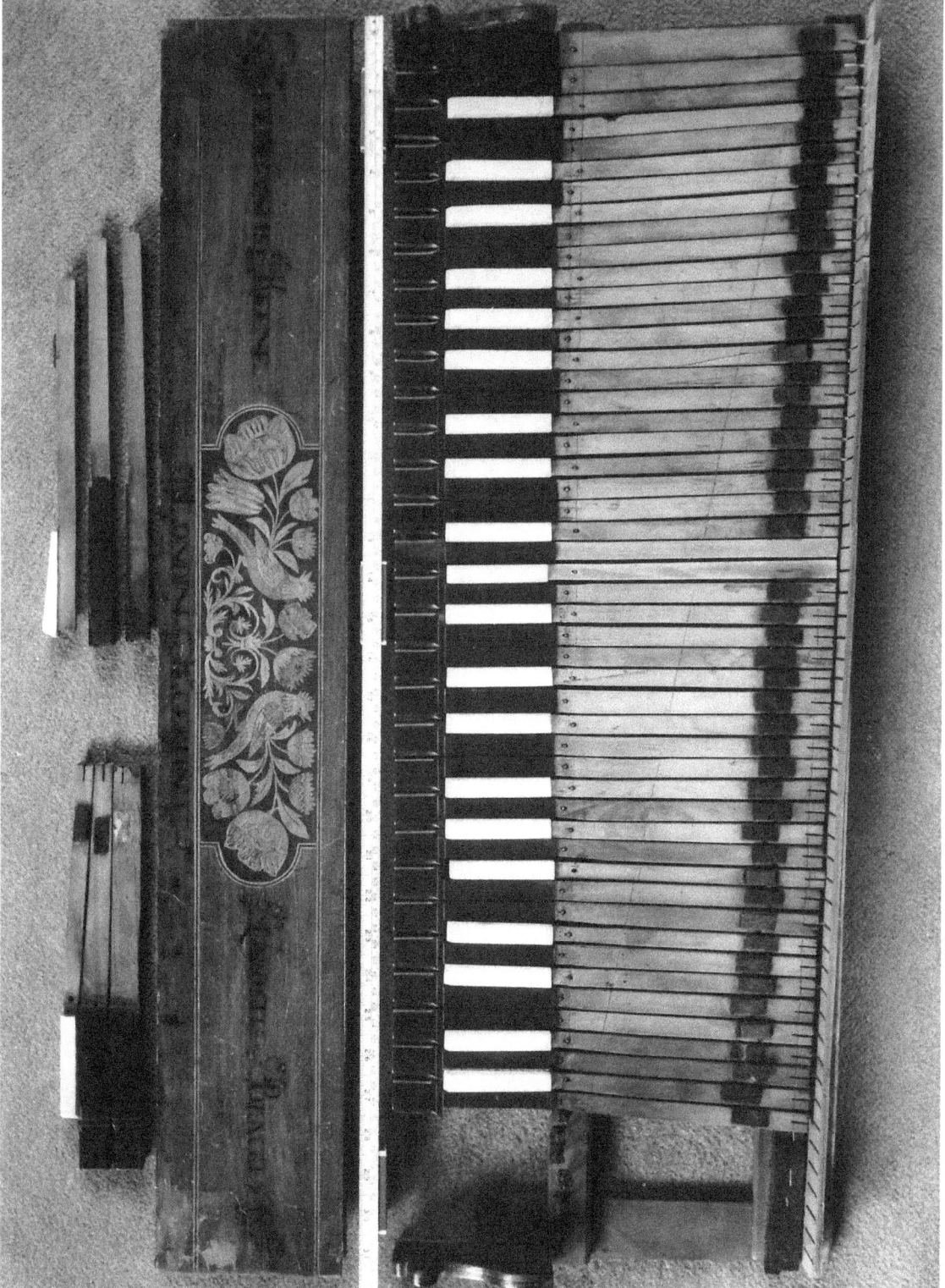

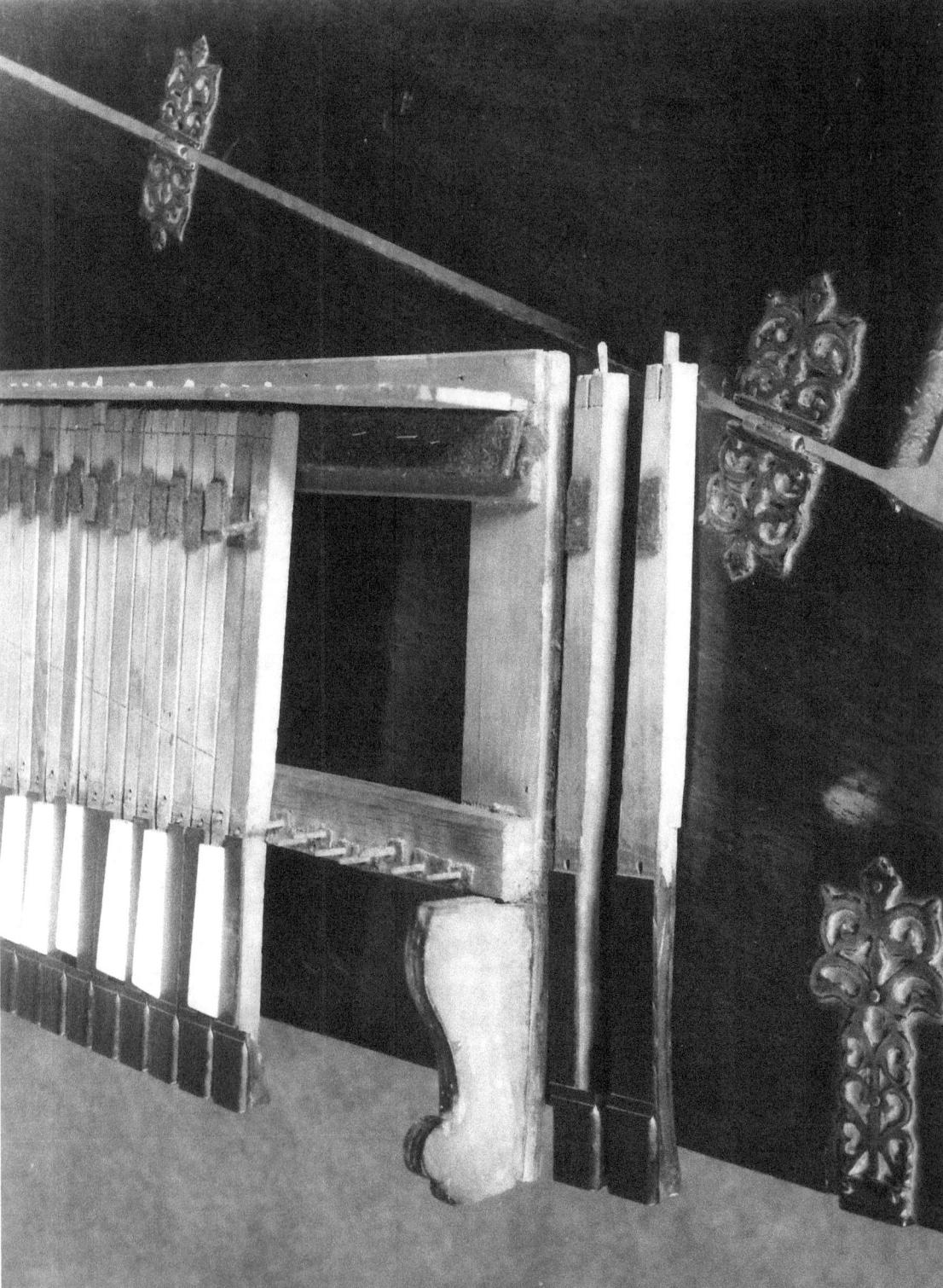

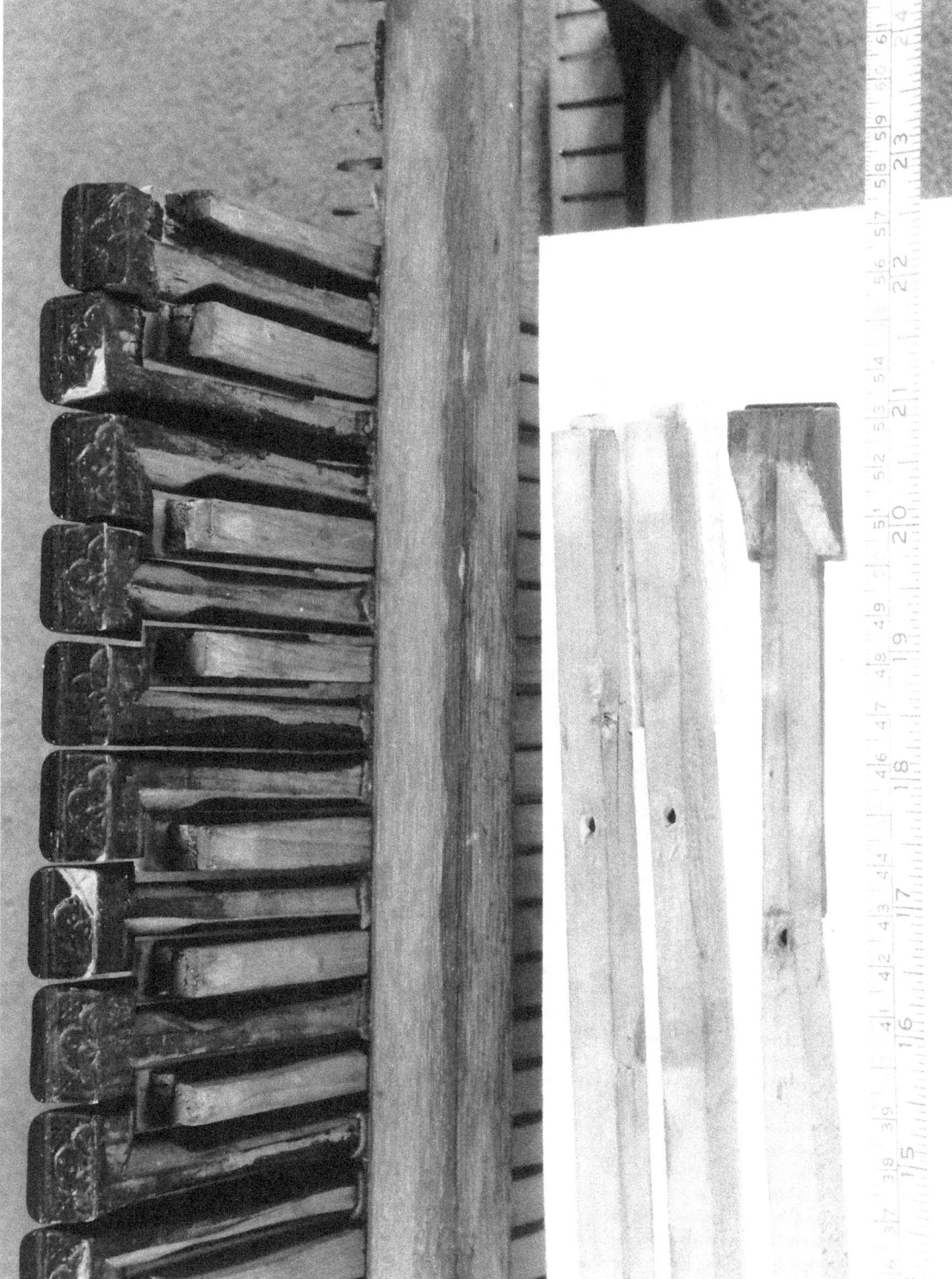

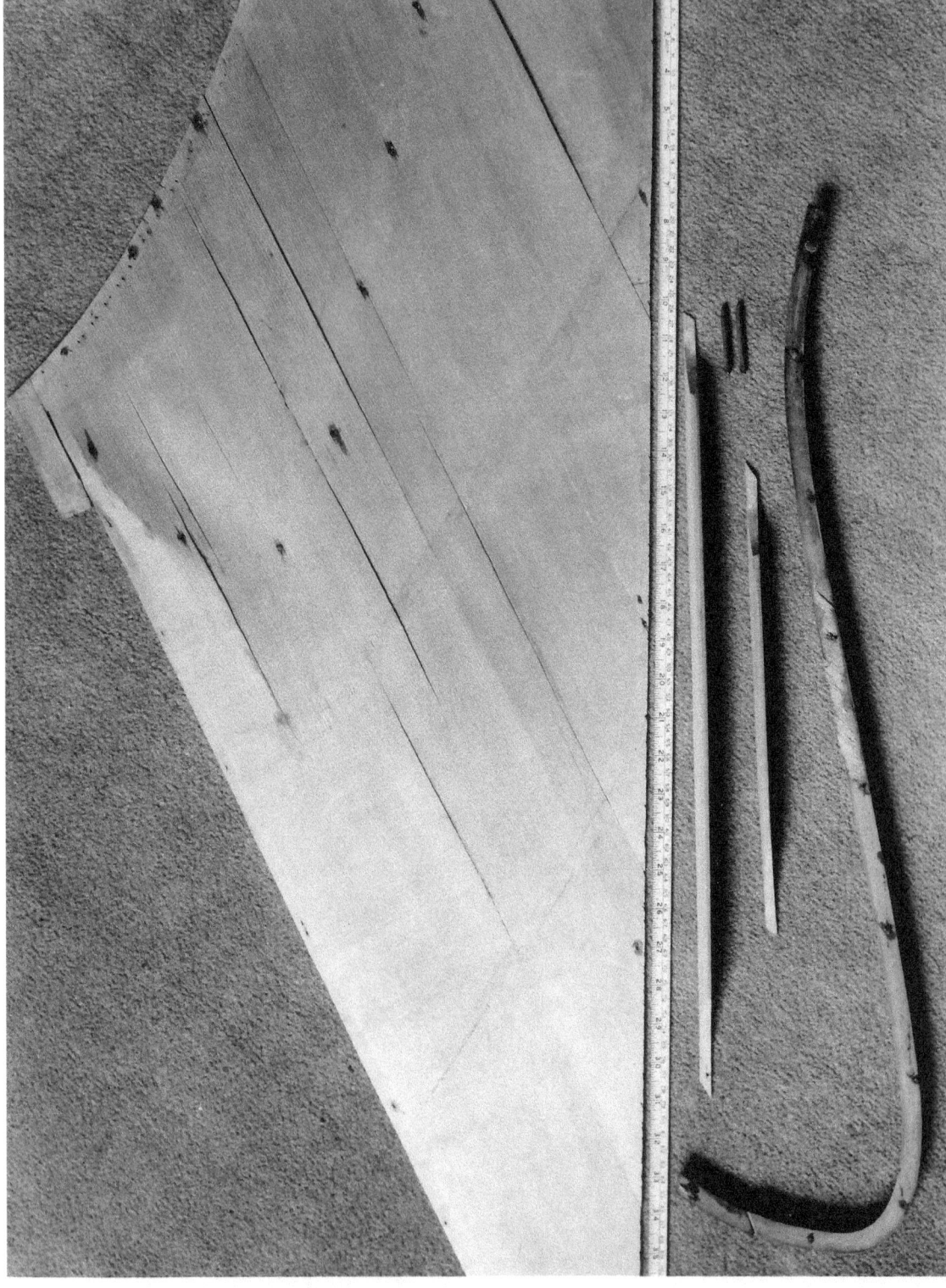

INDEX

Adlung, Jakob, 47
back, fitting, 14
back touch cloth, 23
balance cloth, 23
balance pins
  holes for, 24
  position of, 20, 21
bars, gluing to soundboard, 29
baseboard, 6–8
  assembling, 6
  construction lines on, 8
  cutting out, 8
  gluing, 7
  thicknessing, 7
Bedos de Celles, Dom, 17
bending jig, 5
bentside
  making, 5–6
  fitting, 15
Blanchets, trough owned by, 5
braces, fitting to baseboard, 12
bridge, making & fixing, 27–9
bridge pins, 28
case sides
  cut from one plank, 16
  order of fitting, 14, 15
  when veneered, 15, 30
construction, order of, 2
construction lines
  can be decorative, 19
  not removed, 2
corner blocks, where used, 15, 16
cross planing, 7
crossbanding, 30
dampers, 47–8
diagonal line, use of, 20, 31
Diderot, Denis, 34, 47
ebony for keytops, 17
errors, compensating for, 2–3
flap, when cut, 16
front touch, 46
gauge, soundboard, 27
glue, types of, 3
guide tongues
  fitting, 24
  marking slots for, 20

Haward, spinet jack guide, 9
hitchpin rail, when glued, 30
Hubbard, Frank, 5, 17, 34, 47
jack guide
  how fitted to wrestplank, 12
  how made, 9–11
  slots, octave span of, 11
  tilt of, 11
  types, 9
jackrail
  cloth for, 48
  height of, 48
jacks, 31–8
  adjusting length, 46
  bristle holes in, 35–6
  clearances, 34
  construction lines on, 31
  direction of travel, 12
  dummy, 20
  jamming, 12
  lead weights in, 31–2
  pearwood blocks for 31
  thicknessing, 32–4
  tongues for, 36–8
  tongue slots in, 34–5
  to remove tongue from, 38
  wood used for, 31
jigs, practicality of, 2
joints, shot, 6–7
Keene's spinet, observations on
  back touch cloth, 23
  balance cloth, fitting, 23
  baseboard, scribed lines on, 8
  bentside, tapered, 5
  braces
    fixing to baseboard, 12
    glue runs on, 13
  bridge
    fixing to soundboard, 28
    joint in, 27
    pin position marks on, 28
    pins, tops of filed, 29
    scribed lines round, 28
  case sides
    glue runs on, 16
    use of grain on sides, 16

Keene's spinet – case sides *cont.*
    veneering, 15, 30
  cross planing, 7
  glue, animal, 3
  hitchpin rail, fixing, 30
  jack guide, 9, 10
    slots, not cleaned up, 10
  key-block, bass, line on, 48
  keys
    finishing, 24
    fixing guide tongues, 24
    gluing cloth to 24
    hardwoods for tops, 17
    ivory for sharps, 24
    scribed lines on, 19, 20–1
  lettering on nameboard, 48
  liners, fixing
    to back, 14
    to jack guide, 12
    to tail & bentside, 16
  nameboard, tapered, 33
  nut
    fixing, 40
    line scribed on, 40
    line scribed round, 40
  rack, marking out, 21–2
  rack slots, cutting, 22
  saw
    for cutting keys, 23
    for marquetry, 48
  scale, 39
  shaving blaze not used, 30
  soundboard
    mouldings, 30
    thinner than average, 25
  tuning pins, placing, 41–2
  VV mark, 14
  wrestplank
    fixing to braces, 12, 13
keyboard, 17–21, 23–4
  marking out, 17, 19–21
  saw for cutting, 23–4
keyframe
  assembling & fitting, 17
  locating bars for, 15
keys, *see also* keyboard, 11, 24
keytops, 17, 19, 24
knife used in marking out, 2
lettering *see* nameboard

lid, when to cut, 16
liners, fitting,
  to back, 14
  to jack guide, 12
  to tail and bentside, 16
lockboard, *see* flap
marking out, methods of, 2
marquetry panel, 48
note names, how written, 3
nut, 40
nut pins, 3, 40–1
over-plucking, 45
quilling, 45–6
quills
  angle of, 38
  oiling, 47
  thicknesses of, 47
  types of, 45
rack, 21–3
  cutting slots in, 22
  fitting to keyframe, 23
  marking out, 21, 22
ruler, 2
  keyboard, 17, 19
scale, 39–40
snakewood for keytops, 17
soundboard, 25–7, 29–30
  gauge for, 27
  gluing in, 29–30
  grain direction of, 25
  jointing, 25, 26
  thicknessing, 27
Sprengel, Peter, 5
stringing, 39–45
  starting on top notes, 43
strings
  gauges of, 44
  lengths of, 39–40
  making loops in, 42–3
  safety factor of, 39
tuning pins
  holes for, 42
  making, 41
  positions of, 41–2
  winding wire on, 43–4
variations, random, 2
voicing, 46–7
wrestplank, 9
  fitting to braces, 12–13

www.ingramcontent.com/pod-product-compliance
Lightning Source LLC
LaVergne TN
LVHW081355060426
835510LV00013B/1837